THE DIABETIC BIBLE

Dana Armstrong, R.D., C.D.E.,

Allen Bennett King, M.D., F.A.C.P., F.A.C.E, C.D.E.

pil

Publications International, Ltd.

Dana Armstrong, R.D., C.D.E., received her degree in nutrition and dietetics from the University of California, Davis, and the University of Nebraska Medical Center, Omaha. In private practice for 20 years, she has developed an educational program that has benefited more than 5,000 patients with diabetes. She is cofounder and program director of the Diabetes Care Center in Salinas, California. She specializes in the use of insulin pumps and continuous-glucose-sensing technology (and speaks nationally on these topics) as well as a patient-centered approach to diabetes treatment. Having a child with diabetes, she combines her professional knowledge with personal experience and understanding.

Allen Bennett King, M.D., F.A.C.P., F.A.C.E, C.D.E., received his degrees and training at the University of California, Berkeley; Creighton University Medical School; the University of Colorado; and Stanford University. He has authored more than 50 papers in medical science and speaks nationally on new advances in diabetes care. During his 30 years of practice he has seen more than 10,000 patients with diabetes, some for more than 25 years. He is an assistant clinical professor at the University of California Natividad Medical Center; cofounder and medical director of the Diabetes Care Center in Salinas, California; and son of Earle King, who died in 1978 from complications of diabetes.

In October 1998, Armstrong and King together opened a private practice focused on the treatment, education, and support of people with diabetes. Their philosophy is to empower the patient who has diabetes with the knowledge and education that lets the patient control their health, life, and future.

ISBN-13: 978-1-4127-1003-9
ISBN-10: 1-4127-1003-0

Library of Congress Control Number: 2004094477

This book is for informational purposes and is not intended to provide medical advice. Neither the Editors of Consumer Guide® and Publications International, Ltd., nor the authors or publisher take responsibility for any possible consequences from any treatment, procedure, exercise, dietary modification, action, or application of medication or preparation by any person reading or following the information in this book. The publication of this book does not constitute the practice of medicine, and this book does not attempt to replace your physician or other health care provider. Before undertaking any course of treatment, the authors, editors, and publisher advise the reader to check with a physician or other health care provider.

The brand-name products mentioned in this book are trademarks or service marks of their respective companies. The mention of any product in this book does not constitute an endorsement by the respective proprietors of Publications International, Ltd., nor does it constitute an endorsement by any of these companies that their products should be used in the manner recommended by this book.

All recipes and photographs that contain specific brand names are copyrighted by those companies and/or associations, unless otherwise specified.

Some of the food products listed in this publication may be in limited distribution.

Nutritional Analysis: Linda R. Yoakam, M.S., R.D., L.D.

The nutritional information that appears with each recipe was submitted in part by the participating companies and associations. Every effort has been made to check the accuracy of these numbers. However, because numerous variables account for a wide range of values for certain foods, nutritive analyses in this book should be considered approximate.

Photo credits:

© **Corbis:** Pat Doyle (page 40); Jose Luis Pelaez, Inc. (page 56); David Raymer (page 61); **SuperStock:** Raymond Forbes (page 28); Shaffer/Smith (page 112).

All food photographs *except* that on page 157 copyright © Publications International, Ltd.

Pictured on the front cover *(clockwise from top right):* Fresh Strawberry Cream Pie *(page 292),* Sassy Chicken & Peppers *(page 248),* and Grilled Mozzarella & Roasted Red Pepper Sandwich *(page 222).*

Pictured on the back cover *(bottom left to right):* Sweet and Sour Carrots *(page 270)* and Chocolate Chip Cookies *(page 286).*

Microwave Cooking: Microwave ovens vary in wattage. Use the cooking times as guidelines and check for doneness before adding more time.

Preparation/Cooking Times: Preparation times are based on the approximate amount of time required to assemble the recipe before cooking, baking, chilling, or serving. These times include preparation steps such as measuring, chopping, and mixing. The fact that some preparation and cooking can be done simultaneously is taken into account. Preparation of optional ingredients and serving suggestions is not included.

contents

have you heard the good news?

You don't have to be a prisoner of diabetes, living a life of deprivation, sitting there waiting for complications to develop. By understanding your disease, actively participating in your care, using the management tools at your disposal, and expanding and improving the choices you make every day, you'll feel better and enjoy improved health and tighter diabetes control. You'll also lower your risk of diabetes complications. It takes dedication on your part; the right diabetes care team, with you as captain; and a treatment plan developed especially for you that evolves with your disease. *The Diabetic Bible* is the perfect complement to these, always at hand to explain the what, why, and how of successful diabetes management.

The book's first section is a refresher course on diabetes; its causes, types, and symptoms; how it begins and progresses; and what complications and other medical conditions are associated with it. You'll even learn about the disease's growing incidence in children and whether your family members may be at increased risk.

The second part covers the many tools for managing diabetes, from blood sugar testing and lifestyle changes to pills and insulin. And if you use insulin, the chapter on hypoglycemia (low blood sugar) is a must read.

In the third section, you'll discover that the strict diabetes diet of old has been replaced by options galore, and you have the power to please your tastebuds as you tighten your control. You'll find help with day-to-day dietary decisions that can reign in blood sugar, blood pressure, blood cholesterol, and excess pounds. You'll even find a nutrient counter that lists the calorie, carbohydrate, fiber, total and saturated fat, cholesterol, protein, and sodium contents of hundreds of foods so you can plan meals and determine how foods will affect your blood sugar levels.

The final surprise: more than 100 scrumptious diabetic recipes. Each recipe comes with nutritional information to help you predict how the dish will affect your blood sugar. Mix and match them to create flavorful, exciting meals that fit into your meal plan and help you meet your goals.

The Diabetic Bible makes it easy to say *no* to dieting and deprivation and *yes* to taking control of your diabetes and your life.

educate yourself

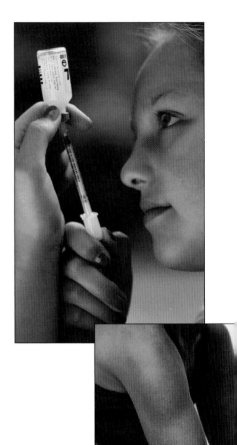

Whether you've only recently learned you have diabetes or you have been battling high blood glucose for years, it never hurts to remind yourself what the fuss is all about. Here, in the first part of the book, you'll rediscover what goes wrong when diabetes develops, why it happens (and why the "adult type" is starting to occur more often in children), what you need to do about it, which other health concerns (including the mysterious-sounding Syndrome X) often accompany diabetes, and what complications are likely to occur if you don't manage your diabetes properly. The more you know and understand about your diabetes, the better prepared you will be to take the steps necessary to keep it under control and prevent its devastating effects.

what is diabetes, anyway?

To get the most from the latest advances and proven treatments in diabetes care, you need to understand just what it means to have diabetes. A good place to start is learning how the body uses fuel and how that process goes awry in diabetes.

getting to know glucose

Even if you've only recently been diagnosed with diabetes, you've probably already heard the term *glucose*. It is an important player in the body and in diabetes.

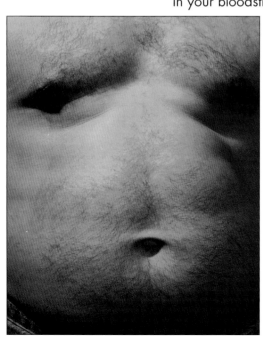

In your bloodstream, circulating to all your organs, is sugar. Most of the sugar in your body is the kind called glucose. (Others include *fructose,* the sugar also found in fruit, and *ribose,* a sugar that makes up the chromosomes that carry your genetic information.) Glucose's main job is to supply the body with energy. The body breaks down

glucose, releasing energy, water, and carbon dioxide.

Glucose is a quickly available fuel used by nearly all tissues in the body. And it's the *only* fuel your brain can use. The brain can survive without glucose for only a short time. Therefore, your brain directs your body to protect your glucose level, making sure it does not fall too low. It's glucose that is meant when people talk about blood sugar, and it is the glucose level in your blood that is affected by diabetes.

The other fuel the body uses are *fatty acids.* Fatty acids differ from glucose in that they provide a source of fuel called upon only during longer periods of fasting. Fatty acids come from the fat we eat and are stored in our fat cells as *triglycerides.* The more fatty acids we store in our fat cells, the more "visible" our energy reserves become.

getting glucose where it needs to go

The glucose in your body comes from three major nutrients: fat, protein, and carbohydrate. About 10 percent of the fat and 50 percent of the protein you eat is eventually broken down into glucose (the rest is used for other purposes or stored in the body's fat cells), but nearly 100 percent of the carbohydrate you eat is broken down into glucose. Chewing and swallowing begins the digestive process of breaking down starches and larger sugar molecules to glucose. The enzymes in your mouth and your intestines complete the breakdown. The glucose is then absorbed into the bloodstream and travels throughout the body.

This process requires help from your *pancreas.* The pancreas is a fist-size organ just behind your stomach. One of its jobs is to make enzymes for food digestion. But the pancreas also plays another important role. It contains small groups of cells, the *islets of Langerhans,* that make hormones, which are released into your bloodstream. Some 80 percent of these islet cells are *beta cells* that make a small protein molecule—the hormone *insulin.*

Insulin plays many important roles in the body, but its primary task is to cause body tissues to take in proteins, fatty acids, and glucose. Insulin is like a key that opens a door to the body's cells, so the nutrients needed by the cells can get inside. When a person who does not have diabetes eats any food, their blood glucose level rises; the beta cells detect this rise and release more insulin. The insulin goes to the liver, telling the liver to make less glucose, and to the muscles and fat

cells, telling them to take up more glucose. This allows nutrients from the recently eaten food to enter and "feed" the body's cells, it keeps blood glucose from rising too high even after eating, and it allows the glucose level to return to a normal, healthy range quickly. When that same healthy person fasts, such as between meals or during sleep, the insulin levels fall, causing the liver to make more glucose to provide energy until the next meal.

In the person with diabetes, this feedback process doesn't work properly. Insulin does not do its job. And the amount of glucose in the blood rises.

detecting diabetes

In a person without diabetes, the body keeps the *plasma glucose level* (see "What's *Plasma?*" on page 10) between meals in the range of 70 to 99 *milligrams per deciliter (mg/dl).* After eating, the glucose level rises, depending on the size and content of the meal, but does not exceed 139 mg/dl. It also quickly returns to the fasting, or between-meal, range.

In a person with diabetes, the blood glucose level rises abnormally high after eating, takes much longer to come down, and doesn't return to the normal range, even during periods of

What's plasma?

Throughout this book, when we refer to blood glucose level, we're referring to the plasma glucose level. The term *plasma* simply refers to the liquid part of the blood that remains after the blood cells have been removed. It's the portion of the blood that is tested during glucose tests in the laboratory or doctor's office. And the difference between blood glucose and plasma glucose is really only important when choosing and reading personal glucose meters, which are discussed in the chapter Monitoring Your Glucose.

fasting. Therefore, to determine if you have diabetes, a doctor must test your blood glucose levels.

There are three different tests available to determine if you have diabetes. The most commonly used is a blood test in which your *fasting plasma glucose* is measured. A fasting test is done more than eight hours after you have had anything to eat or drink. When your fasting plasma glucose is more than 125 mg/dl on two consecutive occasions, diabetes is diagnosed.

Another method is a *random blood glucose test,* which is done without regard to meals. If your random glucose is 200 mg/dl or higher and you have symptoms of diabetes—frequent urination, excessive thirst, excessive hunger, weight loss, or fatigue—the diagnosis of diabetes is made.

The third test is an *oral glucose tolerance test.* This test is done when a test of the fasting plasma glucose shows a level close to normal but diabetes is suspected (because, for example, the above-mentioned symptoms are present). An oral glucose tolerance test is given after three days of a diet high in starches and sugars. After an overnight fast, you arrive at the lab for a two-hour test. Your blood is drawn to measure your fasting plasma level. You are then asked to drink a liquid with a high glucose concentration over a 15-minute period. During the remainder of the test period,

your blood is drawn at specified intervals. It is important to sit for the entire test and report if you feel ill during the test. Diabetes is diagnosed if the blood drawn at the second-hour mark indicates that your blood glucose level is more than 199 mg/dl.

You may have noticed that there's a gap between a glucose level that's considered normal and one that indicates diabetes. A normal fasting glucose level, for example, is less than 100 mg/dl, but it's only when the fasting glucose level rises above 125 mg/dl that a diagnosis of diabetes is made. Likewise, at the end of a two-hour glucose tolerance test, a normal glucose level should be less than 140 mg/dl, and yet a diagnosis of diabetes isn't made unless the glucose level after those two hours is 200 mg/dl or higher. What about the range in between?

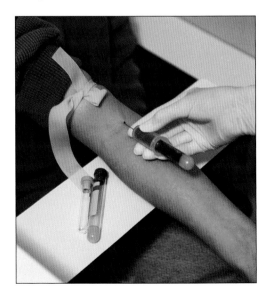

Glucose levels of 100 to 125 mg/dl when fasting and two-hour glucose levels of 140 to 199 mg/dl are not considered diabetes but are not normal, either. People with these levels are diagnosed as having *impaired fasting glucose* and *impaired glucose tolerance* respectively. Although not yet considered to have diabetes, these people have an 11 percent chance of developing diabetes each subsequent year and also have a higher incidence of heart disease.

different kinds of diabetes

Once the diagnosis is made, the next task is to determine what type of diabetes you have. There are three major types of diabetes: type 1 diabetes, type 2 diabetes, and gestational diabetes. Each type of diabetes requires a different treatment approach.

type 1 diabetes

Type 1 diabetes affects about 5 percent of all people who have diabetes. It is sometimes referred to as *juvenile diabetes,* because there is a higher rate of diagnosis in children between the ages of 10 and 14, but people of any age can develop type 1 diabetes. It may also be called *insulin-dependent diabetes,* because diabetes pills are ineffective in treating the high blood glucose level; these individuals require injections of insulin to control their blood glucose. (As you will learn shortly, a small number of people with type 1 who are in the very earliest stages of the disease may not yet require insulin; eventually, however, they will.)

Type 1 diabetes is a disease of "confused" white blood cells. Normally, white blood cells are responsible for recognizing foreign objects in our

making the diagnosis

type of test:	fasting blood glucose (fbg)	random blood glucose (rbg)	oral glucose tolerance
It is **diabetes** when:	FBG > 125 mg/dl on two consecutive blood tests	RBG ≥ 200 mg/dl, plus diabetes symptoms	2-hour glucose level ≥ 200 mg/dl
It is **impaired fasting glucose** when:	FBG ≥ 100 mg/dl and <126 mg/dl		
It is **impaired glucose tolerance** when:			2-hour glucose level is ≥140 mg/dl and < 200 mg/dl
It is **normal** when:	FBG <100 mg/dl		< 140 mg/dl

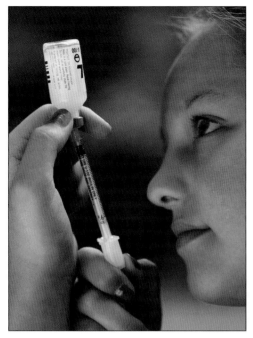

blood and then attacking these foreign objects with antibodies. In type 1 diabetes, the white cells believe the beta cells of the pancreas do not belong there. An inflammation ensues, and the antibodies attack the beta cells. This destruction of beta cells can happen either very quickly or slowly over a long period of time. When enough beta cells are lost, insulin deficiency develops and blood glucose levels begin to rise. Occasionally a viral infection can be identified as the trigger that set off this attack, but generally no such illness can be identified. To make things more complicated, it is not always possible to identify the presence of antibodies (the sign of an autoimmune reaction) in the blood. This is especially common in African and Chinese Americans. In these racial groups, and in some other groups of people, there is probably another cause for the malfunctioning of the beta cells, but this reason has not yet been discovered.

In type 1 diabetes, there is a chance of developing *ketoacidosis* because of the extreme lack of insulin. The lack of enough insulin makes it hard for the body to use glucose for energy. If the body cannot get glucose from the blood, it breaks down fat to supply energy to the cells. One of the products of this breakdown are *ketones,* compounds that are more acidic than normal body tissues; these acidic compounds then accumulate in the blood. Normally ketones are removed from the blood by the kidneys and passed out of the body in urine. When more ketones are produced than the kidneys can handle, excess ketones build up in the blood. If not treated, this can lead to ketoacidosis, an extremely serious and life-threatening condition. This situation may lead to diabetic coma and death.

Your diabetes is most likely type 1 if you develop the disease before age 35, have a lean build, do not have a family history of diabetes, and require insulin injections. Additional tests may be done to confirm the diagnosis. These tests include measuring islet-cell antibodies (the antibodies directed toward destroying the islet cells), the C-peptide level (a measurement of the amount of insulin being made by the body), and urine ketones. A positive islet-cell antibody test, a low C-peptide level, or the presence of ketones in the urine all suggest a diagnosis of type 1 diabetes.

If you have type 1 diabetes, you will probably require insulin to control your glucose. However, on occasion, a person in the earliest stages of type 1 may still have some islet cells left that secrete enough insulin so that insulin injections are not yet required. Pills or changes in diet, activity, and lifestyle may be enough to control blood glucose. Still, because the person has type 1 diabetes, their white blood cells will continue to attack the islet cells, and the remaining insulin-making beta cells will be destroyed. So, with time, insulin injections will become necessary.

type 2 diabetes

Type 2 diabetes is the most common form of diabetes. It is estimated that up to 90 percent of the people who have diabetes have type 2. The cause appears to be resistance to insulin's action and/or a deficiency of insulin secretion. But how does one separate it from type 1 diabetes? Type 2 diabetes almost never causes ketoacidosis and shows no evidence of autoimmunity (in other words, there are no signs of antibodies attacking the islet cells).

People with type 2 diabetes are usually over 35, are overweight, and have a family history of diabetes treated with diet or pills. Separating type 1 and type 2 can be very difficult. Indeed, it has been found that almost 5 percent of adults who are diagnosed as having type 2 actually have type 1. Furthermore, the incidence of type 2 diabetes in childhood is rapidly increasing in frequency, making the automatic diagnosis of type 1 in children with diabetes less reliable as well.

Type 2 diabetes begins decades before diagnosis, with an increasing resistance to insulin. This increasing resistance is the result of genetics, weight gain (especially abdominal fat), decreased activity, and aging. The major site of insulin resistance is the muscle tissue, which normally uses more than 80 percent of the glucose taken into the body. Because of this resistance, the body's insulin levels actually begin to increase. To make up for the lack or

What type of diabetes do I have?

characteristics	type of diabetes	
	1	2
Age of onset	Younger than 35	Older than 35
Need insulin	yes	no
Family history of diabetes	infrequent	usually
Big belly	no	yes
Ketones in urine	yes	no

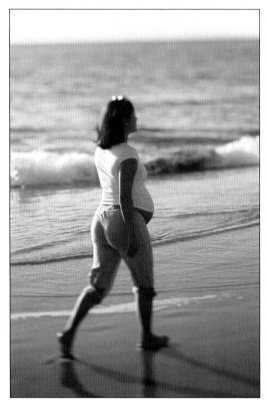

diminished effectiveness of insulin, the body cranks up insulin production. For reasons not entirely clear, in people destined for diabetes, the beta cells slowly fail to keep up with the demand for insulin. They get burned out, in a sense. At first, the plasma glucose level begins to rise above normal after meals; eventually, fasting glucose levels begin to remain above normal, too. When glucose rises high enough to produce symptoms, or when a complication, such as a heart attack, sends the patient to the hospital, the diagnosis of type 2 diabetes is made.

gestational diabetes

Gestational diabetes is diabetes diagnosed for the first time during pregnancy. It occurs in about 3 percent of all pregnancies. Gestational diabetes is diagnosed using a three-hour glucose tolerance test. If any two of the glucose readings during the test exceed the upper limits of normal, the diagnosis is made. Rarely are the glucose levels high enough to harm the mother. The problem is the mother's blood glucose flows into the fetus's blood. The fetus then releases insulin from its pancreas to lower its glucose levels. This forces glucose into the fetus's tissues, causing it to become large for its gestational age and resulting in a difficult labor and delivery.

Throughout the pregnancy, the mother's insulin resistance and glucose levels increase, right up to delivery. With delivery of the baby and placenta, however, the mother's glucose levels promptly return to normal in 97 percent of cases.

Many women with gestational diabetes can control their glucose levels during pregnancy through diet and exercise. Some, however, require insulin shots to keep glucose levels within a healthy range for the baby. New studies have shown that a pill to lower glucose in pregnancy works as well as insulin, but more studies are needed before it is widely accepted.

Women who have had gestational diabetes have a significantly greater chance of developing diabetes sometime in the future, at a general rate of about 3 percent each year. A few studies have shown weight control and increased physical activity may lessen the risk of future diabetes by 50 percent. There are even studies currently under way to evaluate the ability of some of the new diabetes pills to prevent diabetes in women who have had gestational diabetes.

will my kids get diabetes?

About 20 percent of Americans 40 to 75 years of age have diabetes, and about half don't even know it. Certain ethnic groups have an even higher incidence of diabetes; these include African, Asian, and Hispanic Americans; Pacific Islanders; and Native Americans. Indeed, in some Native American tribes, eight of every ten tribe members have diabetes. Further, the prevalence of diabetes in the United States is increasing due to the aging of the population, the change in ethnic mix toward a greater percentage of susceptible people, increasing obesity, and decreasing physical activity.

Type 2 diabetes is inherited as a dominant trait. If you have type 2 diabetes, each one of your children has approximately a one-in-three, or a bit above a 30 percent, chance of developing it, too. People who have type 2 usually have some relative who also has the disease. But contrary to popular myth, diabetes does not skip generations. (You'll find more information on diabetes and heredity in the chapter Children and Diabetes.)

why control glucose?

When your blood glucose rises into the 140 to 180 mg/dl range, it begins to cause damage throughout your body, although you may not notice symptoms until it hovers above 180. The excess glucose begins to spill over into your urine, causing increased urination; and, because you're losing more water through increased urination, you have increased thirst. Because your body's cells can't take in and use the glucose in your blood, they become starved for fuel; you feel hungry and fatigued and become unusually sleepy, especially after a meal. If your glucose levels remain elevated, your white blood cells don't work as well, leaving you more vulnerable to infections. Wounds become slow to heal, and you are more likely to get bladder and yeast infections. If your glucose levels stay above normal, the glucose becomes increasingly toxic to your body, and severe damage begins to occur in your eyes, kidneys, feet, and heart.

That's only a brief description of the changes that untreated diabetes can cause in your body (you'll find more details in Diabetes Complications and Long-Term Concerns). But you can take steps to forestall such frightening consequences of high blood glucose. Managing your diabetes wisely and well means getting control not only of your blood glucose but of your life. You need to become educated about diabetes, you need to pay more attention to what is happening in your body and your life, and you need to start living in awareness. In other words, you need to take charge.

Factors that increase your risk of developing diabetes

- You are overweight, especially if you have a lot of abdominal fat.
- You get little or no exercise.
- You are 45 years of age or older.
- You are a woman who has given birth to a baby weighing more than nine pounds.
- You have a sister, brother, or parent who has diabetes.
- You are an African American, Hispanic American, Asian American, or Native American or are a Pacific Islander.

taking command of your care

The latest approach to diabetes treatment puts you in charge. You become the boss of your diabetes team, choosing the staff that best serves your needs, tracking your progress, and keeping your eyes on the ultimate goal—your health and well-being.

assemble your staff

Getting the best treatment is not simply a matter of keeping your doctor's appointments and taking pills. Diabetes affects many aspects of your life. And since nobody knows your life better than you do, you must step into the role of the "general" of your diabetes care team in order to get your treatment needs met.

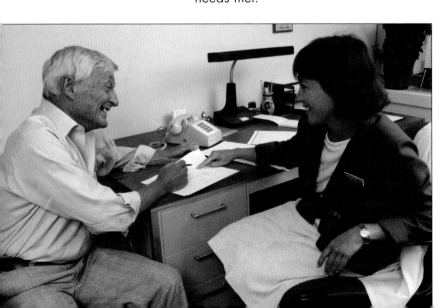

As the general, you'll want to surround yourself with knowledgeable, trustworthy, expert advisors—your diabetes care team—who can help you get the information, advice, treatments, and support you need to manage your diabetes effectively. This team may include your doctor, diabetes educator, dietitian, pharmacist, and dentist. Also onboard may be a mental-health professional, an eye doctor, a podiatrist (foot doctor), and a cardiologist (heart specialist). As you go about assembling your team, remember that these people work for *you*. You are hiring them to help you learn about diabetes, understand how it specifically affects you, and provide you with the tools that let you make your own informed health care decisions.

Your first task is to find a doctor. You'll not only want a physician who has skill and experience in diagnosing and treating diabetes, but also one who will support and work with you in becoming your own diabetes general. Together you and your doctor need to develop a good working relationship where there is mutual understanding, respect, and trust. You will need to feel comfortable talking with and asking questions of your doctor. If you are unable to develop such a relationship, you need to find another doctor.

There are many diabetes specialists, and you can get a list of the doctors in your area by contacting the American Diabetes Association, or ADA (at www.diabetes.org or 1-800-DIABETES). You can also call your local medical society and ask for a list of doctors who are "board certified" in endocrinology (the specialty that focuses on hormonal disorders, such as diabetes), internal medicine, or family practice. If you cannot find a specialist near you, pick a primary care doctor who will work with you and who will not hesitate to refer you to a specialist when one might be needed.

Education is by far the most basic tool of diabetes care. It involves learning how to take care of yourself and your diabetes, and it brings you into the decision-making process for your own health. So after you find a doctor, you'll need to add a diabetes educator to your team. The diabetes educator will provide you with information and one-on-one guidance. As with your doctor, the educator you choose should be someone you feel comfortable talking to and feel you can contact with questions about the practical details of diabetes care.

Most often, a diabetes educator will also be a nurse, dietitian, or pharma-cist by training. If possible, choose a certified diabetes educator, or CDE. A CDE is a trained health professional who is certified by the National Certification Board for Diabetes Educators to teach people with diabetes how to manage the disease. CDEs must have at least two years' and 1,000 hours of experience in diabetes education, be currently employed in a defined role as a diabetes educator for a minimum of four hours each week, and have successfully completed a comprehensive examination covering diabetes. Your physician or health plan may be able to refer you to a certified diabetes educator, or you can contact the American Association of Diabetes Educators (at www.aadenet.org or 1-800-338-3633) for the names of diabetes educators in your area.

With the help of your doctor and diabetes educator, you should be able to get additional referrals to a dentist, eye doctor, podiatrist, and cardiologist if needed. If you already have an established relationship with a dentist or eye doctor, be sure to discuss your diabetes diagnosis with them and perhaps even put them in touch with the other members of your team so that they can collaborate on your care.

focus on taking control

Being diagnosed with diabetes and then being told to alter your life can spark some pretty intense emotions. It's natural to feel stressed, afraid, sad, or even angry at the news that you have this disease. But while such reactions may be normal, they can be harmful if you don't work through them and then refocus your energy into taking care of yourself and your diabetes.

For some people, the stress of a diabetes diagnosis can turn into denial. Regularly testing your blood glucose level simply becomes a constant reminder that you have diabetes. So, you skip the testing in an effort to pretend you don't really have the disease. To further the denial, you attribute your symptoms of high glucose levels, such as excessive thirst and fatigue, to some other cause, such as the hot weather or working long hours. Perhaps you cancel or simply don't show up for your medical appointments. Ignoring the fact that you have diabetes will not make it go away. People who live in denial about their diabetes die.

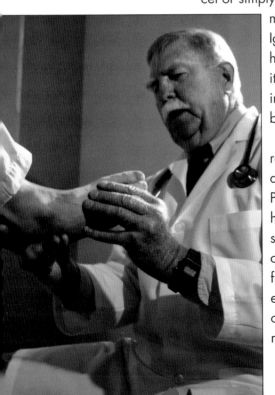

Fear, too, is a common reaction to the stress of dealing with diabetes. Perhaps you know or have heard of someone who is suffering from multiple, crippling complications from diabetes or may have even died of diabetes complications. While it makes sense to fear the complications of diabetes, you need not let that fear paralyze you. Instead, use the fear of diabetes complications as strong motivation for learning all you can about your disease and working hard to gain the best possible control of your glucose levels.

Feeling sad or down is yet another common reaction to a diabetes diagnosis; it can also occur in response to the stress of coping with the disease. When that blue feeling lasts more than a few weeks or really begins to interfere with your daily life or with taking care of your diabetes, it may be depression. Depression is a biochemical condition. It is not a defect in your character. Once this condition is treated with therapy or medications, your mood and functioning will improve.

If you suspect that you may be suffering from depression, you should discuss it with your doctor. Your doctor may choose from many available medications and/or may refer you to a psychotherapist, psychologist, or psychiatrist.

chart your own course

In terms of diabetes care, charting your own course is not just a figure of speech. As the general in charge of your diabetes care, you should create your own care chart, much like the kind a doctor keeps. This way, you can have all the information about your disease in one place, and you can take it with you each time you meet with a member of your diabetes care team.

You'll find a list of the types of information your chart should contain in the box to the right. It is particularly crucial that your chart include a complete, accurate, and up-to-date list of all of your medications and the strength and dose of each. Be sure to include all prescription drugs and any nonprescription medicines, vitamins, minerals, and natural products you take. You may be seeing more than one doctor, and it is important that each one knows what the other has prescribed for you and what over-the-counter products you take so that together you can avoid dangerous interactions. It is also important for *you* to know what you are taking, why you are taking it, and what side effects or warning signs may occur. It is, after all, your body, and you shouldn't put anything in it that you don't understand. Be sure to note in your chart any side effects or unusual symptoms you experience that you suspect may be connected to your medications. This way you can inquire about them the next time you talk to your doctor.

It's also very helpful to keep a running list of questions you have about diabetes so that you can ask your team. Jot them down as they occur to you. Often, under the pressure of limited time

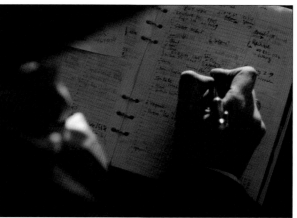

or nervousness during the appointment, you can easily forget questions that otherwise seemed so clear just the day prior. Also, prioritize your questions so the most important questions are answered first. If you aren't able to cover all of your questions during the visit, inform your doctor so that you can make another appointment and get answers to the remainder of your questions.

Take time to prepare for each visit the night prior to the appointment. Be sure to bring your chart as well as your blood glucose meter and any additional log or record books (you'll learn more about meters and log books in upcoming chapters).

Remember, you are the general in charge of your care. Take some time to make sure you have the personnel, focus, and resources at hand to accomplish your mission. That mission—taking care of your diabetes and yourself—really is a matter of life and death.

What to include in your own medical chart:

- List of your medicines; their strengths; how, when, and why you take them; who prescribed them
- List of your medical conditions and dates of diagnosis, any drug allergies, all major medical events and surgeries
- List of all your doctors and health care professionals and their office and emergency phone numbers
- Laboratory test results, handouts, information sheets, and instructions given to you by your diabetes care team
- List of questions you have for your doctor or other diabetes care professional

diabetes complications and long-term concerns

Three keys to treating, delaying, or preventing complications

EDUCATION
Learn as much as you can about diabetes.

EARLY DETECTION
Learn the signs and symptoms of potential problems.

REGULAR OFFICE VISITS
Set up a schedule, and *stick to it!*

It can be hard to face each day knowing you have to test your blood glucose, watch what you eat, keep records, and all the rest. But keeping tight control and taking care of yourself now can help you keep the dreaded long-term complications of diabetes at bay.

the bad news—and the good

People with diabetes are vulnerable to a variety of problems that can develop after they have had the disease for many years. A person with diabetes is more likely than other people to have a heart attack, a stroke, eye problems that can lead to blindness, kidney disease, a foot or leg amputation, frequent infections, and sexual problems. All of these are truly serious long-term problems and are more likely to occur if blood glucose levels have been high over many years.

Fortunately, in this new century, diabetes complications and other problems are no longer inevitable—unless you and your team do not take good care now. People with diabetes can live long, healthful, and productive lives. To do so challenges you and your diabetes care team to become intimately involved in recognizing, treating, and doing whatever it takes to prevent or delay the long-term problems of diabetes.

There are three key areas that will help you to treat, delay, or, better yet, prevent diabetes complications. You need to start with education. Learn the how, what, and why of complications. While these problems may be scary to think about, learning about them can help you take a proactive stance. Next, understand the earliest signs and symptoms of problems. Know your lab-test results and keep track of changes. Any change, even when results are still in the normal range, may indicate that problems might be developing. Finally, make regular office visits with your diabetes care team and keep the appointments, even if you are feeling well. See your team at least every three months when you are doing and feeling well, and contact them immediately if you are having problems. Working together, you and your health professionals will form a strong prevention team.

how do problems start?

When blood glucose levels exceed 140 mg/dl, the glucose becomes toxic to your body. The excess glucose spills over into the urine, causing frequent urination and, consequently, increased thirst. This leads to dehydration, which causes muscle cramps and dizziness. Because glucose is not getting into the cells very well, if at all, your cells can't get the energy they need to function. You feel fatigued and hungry and you may begin to lose weight. In addition, the excess glucose impairs the ability of your white blood cells to fight off infections and heal wounds. Finally, your vision becomes blurry and you experience great fluctuations in your sight. This occurs because glucose has entered the lenses of your eyes. Inside your lenses the glucose is changed to sorbitol. The sorbitol pulls water into the lenses, which causes them to swell. This swelling changes the shape of your lenses, and this affects your vision.

These changes in your body are generally recognized as the "early warning signs" of diabetes, and one or more of these may have even sent you to your doctor in the first place. Early on, all of these problems are completely reversible with the normalization of your glucose levels. It is only when your body is bathed in toxic glucose levels over time that these problems continue and the long-term complications of diabetes develop.

why do problems continue?

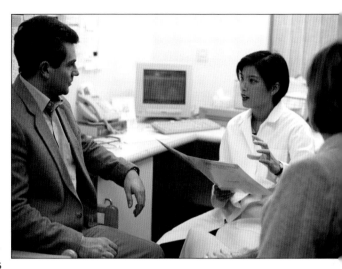

There are two significant events that take place when glucose remains above 140 mg/dl over extended periods of time. The first event is the formation of *advanced glycated end products,* also known as *AGEs,* and the second event is *oxidation.*

Have you ever looked at a freshly baked turkey and noticed how the skin has turned a golden brown and become stiff and crispy? Well, that is an example of glucose combining with protein, in an oven at 350 degrees Fahrenheit, to form advanced glycated end products. In the human body, glucose combines with protein in the same way but is baked at the lower temperature of 98.6 degrees Fahrenheit. The development of these long-lived products occurs in everyone, and they accumulate as we age. For people with diabetes, who have elevated glucose levels, these AGEs form at an accelerated rate. As the AGEs accumulate, the proteins in your body thicken, become brittle, and no longer slip and slide as well. This is the cause of some of the shoulder pain and joint stiffness in people who have poorly controlled diabetes. More seriously, the accumulation of AGEs affects the blood vessels of the kidneys, eyes, feet, and large blood vessels of the body, causing complications.

The other event that occurs at an accelerated rate in diabetes is oxidation. Oxidation is the process that causes rust on cars. Similar damage occurs naturally in the human body. When your body breaks down glucose for energy, byproducts called *free radicals* are made. These free radicals add oxygen to everything in sight, damaging cellular tissue. It is as if your bloodstream and blood vessels are "rusting out." As this "rusting" continues, it damages the linings of your blood vessels and causes various tissues in your body to malfunction. If glucose levels are elevated, high numbers of free radicals are formed and more "rusting," or oxidation, occurs.

seeing after your eyes

Ever wonder how your eyes "see"? You see an object when light is reflected off of it and directed back to your eye. The light enters your eye through a clear covering called the cornea. It passes through the lens, which focuses the light onto the retina, the light-sensing tissue at the back of the eye. The retina translates these visual signals into electrical impulses that are sent, by way of the optic nerve, to the brain so we can "see" the image. The retina is supplied with nutrients and oxygen by tiny blood vessels. If glucose levels are elevated, AGEs and oxidation cause the tiny blood vessels in the retina to thicken in some parts and weaken in others. This leads to the development of diabetic retinopathy, a disease of the blood vessels of the retina of the eye.

As the tiny blood vessels in the retina become swollen, they leak a little fluid into the center of the retina, which may cause your sight to become permanently blurred. This condition is called *background retinopathy*. If the retinopathy progresses, the deterioration of your sight will progress as well. To try to supply the retina with nutrients and oxygen, many new, tiny blood vessels grow out and across the eye. This is called *neovascularization*. These vessels are very fragile and break easily, causing bleeding into the center of your eye, blocking vision and causing blindness. Scar tissue may also form near the retina, pulling it away from the back of the eye. This stage is called *proliferative retinopathy*, and it can lead to impaired vision and even blindness.

Treatment for diabetic retinopathy can help prevent loss of vision and can sometimes restore some lost vision or stop the progression of neovascularization. Thanks to modern medicine and laser technology, neovascularization can be treated. A laser beam can be focused on these fragile blood vessels, causing them to clot and stop bleeding. But this has to be done early in the course of the disease to be effective.

While research is progressing on how to alter blood flow in the eyes to prevent the early changes of diabetic retinopathy, the best form of treatment is prevention. It is now well known that there are two essential things you can do to best safeguard your vision: Control your blood glucose levels, and have regularly scheduled eye exams. Sound medical management of your diabetes by you and your team and regular, yearly eye examinations can all but eliminate retinopathy. What's more, for 95 percent of people with diabetes who are already affected by some abnormal blood-vessel growth, early screening and prompt treatment can prevent blindness.

In addition to retinopathy, people with diabetes can have other eye problems that demand attention. Glaucoma, which is caused by too much pressure in the eye, can occur in anyone and is a problem that is not related to diabetes. However, people with diabetes have a greater risk of developing glaucoma. You may have no symptoms of glaucoma, but it can be diagnosed with a simple test that measures pressure in your eye. If detected, it should be treated promptly. When glaucoma is undetected or left untreated, blindness results, which is yet another reason to have regular eye exams by an eye doctor.

Another common eye problem is a cataract, in which the lens of the eye becomes cloudy. This happens in a lot of people as they get older; however, cataracts are more common in people with diabetes. The cloudy crystals in the lens of the eye are caused in part by AGEs. They can lead to poor night vision and, eventually, blindness if not treated. A cataract is treated by removing the lens and replacing it with an implant. Such surgery is done routinely without complications at surgical centers, and most patients are right back to their usual routine within a day or two.

The latest techniques in modern medicine can indeed help to prevent blindness caused by diabetes. But the key is to catch changes early; that's why regular screening is essential.

keeping your kidneys fit

Your kidneys do many things, but the most important are getting rid of products from your blood by excreting them in urine and maintaining a proper mineral and fluid balance in your body. In this way, your kidneys are a bit like a filter or sieve, keeping the right amounts of the good stuff in and getting rid of the things you don't need.

There are a tremendous number of tiny blood vessels that feed the very small cavities in your kidneys, much like the many tiny blood vessels that feed the tissues in your eyes. The vessels in the kidneys have selective-size pores that allow certain molecules to fall into the cavities and be carried out with the urine while at the same time keeping needed molecules from leaving the body. As your glucose levels remain elevated, AGEs build up in the walls of the blood vessels, ironically causing the vessels to become abnor-

mally porous. In addition to AGEs, high blood pressure, nicotine use, and certain other conditions can damage the small blood vessels of the kidneys. As a result, protein molecules start leaking through the pores in the blood vessels and end up in the urine.

In the early stages of kidney disease, albumin, the major protein in your blood, begins to leak through the damaged vessels and into the urine at an abnormal rate. This condition is called *proteinuria* (or in the earliest

stages, *microalbuminuria,* since only small amounts of protein appear in the urine). Normally, less than 30 micrograms (a microgram, or mcg, is one-millionth of a gram) of albumin are found in your urine on any given day. Results greater than 30 mcg indicate kidney damage.

As kidney disease progresses, the pores in the kidneys' blood vessels become larger due to damage, and more protein is lost. When the protein loss reaches 1,000 milligrams, or 1 gram, each day, you may notice puffiness in your ankles due to fluid buildup (edema). As the kidneys become less effective at filtering, waste products slowly begin to collect in the blood; this buildup can be measured and is called your *serum creatinine level.* As the creatinine level increases, so do the levels of other waste products, causing you to become nauseated and fatigued. The waste buildup poisons the kidneys, harming their ability to make erythropoietin, a substance needed by your bone marrow to make oxygen-carrying red blood cells; you become anemic, which means your body's cells become starved for oxygen. At this point, your kidneys can no longer do their most basic job, and you require dialysis. Dialysis involves being hooked to a machine that removes the wastes from your blood.

But kidney disease and the slow deterioration of your body's filtering system do not need to happen. There are several things you can do to protect your kidneys and reduce the likelihood of kidney problems, prevent current problems from becoming worse, and even reverse problems that have started.

get screened. Maintaining kidney health starts with yearly screening for microalbumin. This test looks for small amounts of protein in the urine that cannot be detected by the usual "dipstick" test done during routine urinalysis. (Note, however, that infection, severe stress, heart failure, or strenuous exercise before the test can also increase levels of protein in your urine.) Should the results show increased microalbumin in your urine, the test needs to be repeated. If the second test is also positive, treatment to return this number to normal should begin.

tighten your control. To keep your kidneys healthy or prevent problems from becoming worse, you need to keep blood glucose tightly controlled. Kidney problems result from an increased glucose load, causing a buildup of AGEs. The closer to normal you keep your glucose levels, the better for your kidneys. With the guidance of your team, strive for an HbA1c (discussed in the chapter HbA1c: Looking Back to Move Forward) of less than 7 percent, or less than 6 percent if that's possible without risking hypoglycemia (low blood glucose).

keep your blood pressure in check. It is important to maintain a normal blood pressure and to check it often. When blood pressure is high (above

130/80 mm Hg), it slowly damages the kidneys. Have your pressure checked often, and learn how to monitor it at home. If it is consistently high, early treatment is important. Nicotine, salt, caffeine, and alcohol all may raise blood pressure. By contrast, adding extra physical activity to your life can help lower your blood pressure.

watch your meds. Make sure you avoid medications that can damage your kidneys. When your doctor chooses a drug for you, such as an antibiotic for infection, confirm that it does not have kidney damage as a possible side effect. Be aware that some over-the-counter drugs can cause problems, too. Excessive use of non-steroidal anti-inflammatory drugs (NSAIDs), such as aspirin and ibuprofen, can cause damage to the kidneys. It is safe to use these once in a while as recommended on the bottle. Large

Take care of your kidneys

- Have a screening test done yearly for microalbumin.
- Improve your blood glucose control.
- Maintain a normal blood pressure.
- Avoid medications that can damage your kidneys.
- Avoid all forms of nicotine.
- Use preventive medications when needed.
- Lower your intake of protein.

daily doses have been associated with kidney problems, however, so if you need to treat ongoing pain or inflammation, talk to your doctor before using large doses of NSAIDs.

say no to nicotine. To maintain the health of your kidneys, you must avoid all forms of nicotine. Nicotine is as harmful to the kidneys as untreated high blood pressure is. Because nicotine is so addictive, the best policy is to never start. If you already smoke or chew tobacco, ask your doctor about resources to help you quit.

take an ACE or ARB. To help slow or reverse kidney disease, it is recommended that prescription medications called *angiotensin converting enzyme (ACE) inhibitors* or *angiotensin receptor blockers (ARBs)* be used when needed. Studies have shown that these classes of blood pressure medicines can slow kidney disease and protect the kidneys from further damage. In addition, they prevent damage to other blood vessels in the body. Started slowly, and taken until there is a change in your kidney status, they will not abnormally lower your blood pressure. If you are already taking a medication for high blood pressure, speak with your doctor and make sure you are on an ACE inhibitor or an ARB.

go easy on protein. Finally, lower the amount of protein in your diet, since it can aggravate kidney problems. When your kidney function

begins to decrease, eating less protein generally helps to slow the process. The protein is an extra load for the kidneys to handle, because the nitrogen from the breakdown of proteins tends to poison the kidneys. For an exact diet prescription to maintain your kidney health, consult your doctor, diabetes educator, and dietitian.

taking care of your tootsies

Diabetes is the most common cause of limb loss, other than accidents, in the United States. Problems begin in your legs or feet due to changes in your blood vessels and nerves; those changes are caused by excess glucose, AGEs, and oxidation. Blood vessels become blocked, and your legs and feet do not receive enough blood. This causes aching pains in your legs and feet, especially when walking, and sores that heal slowly. To compound the problem, your nerves become poisoned by the high levels of glucose, resulting in pain, numbness, and a tingling feeling in your feet and legs, all of which dull the sensitivity of your nerves and your ability to sense a potential problem with your feet. You may not notice a sore caused by a tight, rubbing shoe or a blister from a new pair of shoes. If ignored and left untreated, the sore can become infected and, due to poor blood circulation, the toe or foot may need to be amputated.

Amputation is not an inevitable part of living with diabetes, however. Proper foot care and regular visits to your diabetes care team can prevent foot and leg sores and ensure that any that do appear don't become infected and painful. Proper foot care requires a combined effort by you and your doctor. You need to know what you can do to prevent problems and what to expect from your doctor as well.

Self-care includes the inspection of your feet for sores, cuts, or infection. Get a handheld mirror and examine your feet thoroughly every day. Clean your feet daily and dry them well, especially between the toes, and keep them soft by using lotion after a bath or shower. Each time you buy shoes, have both the width and length of each foot measured to make sure your shoes fit well and have enough space for your toes. Always wear shoes; never go barefoot, even in the home, where you can accidentally kick furniture or step on something sharp hidden in carpeting. If you go to the beach, wear sandals or water socks to protect your feet from sharp objects and pointy rocks in the sand. And finally, never, ever, do bathroom surgery on your feet. Corns, calluses, ingrown toenails, and thick, fungal nails are best left to a podiatrist. A podiatrist can do foot surgery, trim your nails (or teach you how to safely and properly trim them at home), and prescribe medications for

your feet when needed. You need to see a podiatrist regularly if you have lost any sensation in your feet, if you cannot cut your own nails, or if you have a foot ulcer.

It is also your responsibility to assist your team in the care of your feet by being prepared for appointments. Uncover your feet once you're in the examining room. Tell your doctor about any foot-care concerns. Have the doctor inspect all surfaces of your feet, including the soles and between the toes. Make sure your doctor checks the pulses in both feet; this indicates how well the blood is circulating to your feet. Finally, your doctor should do a special test to check the sensation in your feet. If you have lost the protective sensation in your feet, you are vulnerable to infections, sores, and, ultimately, foot loss. This problem alone, or in combination with limited circulation, can potentially spell real trouble. It means you need to take extra precautions to keep your feet safe. And while you cannot always avoid a loss of sensation or decreased circulation in your legs, studies have shown that you have a better chance of avoiding problems if you take good care of your feet, do not smoke, and keep both your blood pressure and diabetes under good control.

diabetes and syndrome X

If you have type 2 diabetes, you more than likely also have Syndrome X. The two together can be deadly unless you take steps to monitor them regularly and keep them both under control.

the discovery

In the mid-1970s, Dr. Gerald Reaven at Stanford University Medical Center described a condition that he coined "Syndrome X." He noted a clustering of medical conditions that were associated with a very high rate of coronary artery disease (a common type of heart disease that affects the blood vessels feeding the heart). These conditions included high blood pressure, glucose intolerance, and high levels of cholesterol and triglycerides in the blood; these, in turn, were associated with insulin resistance and, consequently, high insulin levels. Since the discovery of Syndrome X, there has been a great deal of focus and many studies conducted to try to

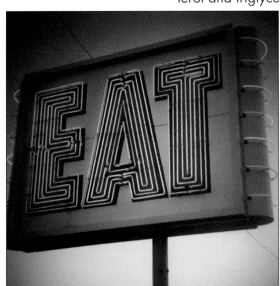

understand what causes it. Some of the resulting fingers of blame point to our ever-expanding waistlines.

the belly connection

Each of us is here today because our ancestors had the genetics that allowed them to survive during times of frequent famine. Back then, if you had a fast metabolism, required a lot of food to maintain your weight, and lost weight readily when food was scarce, you didn't survive. Those that did survive the lean times passed on their genes, and that inheritance is still apparent today. These "thrifty" genes are still helping us conserve calories and are reluctant to let us lose fat stores.

For those of us who live in this land of plenty—a land that's thankfully short on famine but also short on manual labor—these same genes make it difficult to lose extra weight. To compound this effect, if you weighed less than six pounds when you were born, your body chemistry tends to favor conserving fat for the rest of your life. And, of course, there's no ignoring the fact that here in America, the older we get, the less active we tend to become,

which means our fat stores just keep piling up. In people whose fat stores accumulate primarily in the abdominal area, as opposed to the buttocks, hips, and thighs, a widening girth sets the stage for Syndrome X.

where the food goes

When you eat, your food is broken down in your small intestines into three basic nutrients—amino acids, glucose, and fatty acids. From your intestines, the nutrients enter the bloodstream, where they can be picked up and used by the cells that need them.

The cells pluck amino acids from the bloodstream and use them to build a wide array of necessary proteins. In a pinch, the amino acids can also be broken down for energy; some can even be made into glucose. But because of protein's many other important and unique roles, the body generally uses amino acids for energy only when it cannot get enough from carbohydrate and fat. The body does not have a storage form of amino acids; if too many are taken in, the body will break them down, excrete parts of them, and turn the remnants over to be stored as glucose or fatty acids. So when other fuels are not available and the body is forced to call upon amino acids for energy, the body must divert them from their other uses or break down protein that is already in use elsewhere (such as in muscle tissue).

The Food You Eat		
IS MADE UP OF		
Proteins	Carbohydrates	Fats
WHICH ARE THEN BROKEN DOWN IN YOUR GUT INTO		
Amino Acids	Glucose	Fatty Acids
WHICH ARE THEN USED BY THE BODY'S CELLS FOR BASIC FUNCTIONS, BURNED FOR ENERGY, OR, WHEN WE TAKE IN MORE ENERGY THAN WE NEED, STORED AS		
Protein (primarily as part of muscle tissue)	Glycogen (in the muscles)	Triglycerides (in fat cells deep in your abdomen and in surface fat cells found all over the body)

The glucose molecules released during digestion go to the liver and to the cells, where they can be immediately broken down for energy or stored as glycogen. The muscle cells take in the most glucose, which they tend to keep for themselves. The liver also maintains a store of glycogen, which it breaks down into glucose and shares with the brain and other tissues between meals. Glucose is a readily available form of fuel, but because glucose molecules hold a lot of water and so are rather large, the body can only store a limited amount of them.

The fatty acids from a meal also enter the bloodstream and head toward the liver, where they can be picked up and used or stored for energy. The liver packages the fatty acids and sends them out to be used by the cells or stored as triglycerides. These dense packets of fat are the

body's main form of stored energy. Triglycerides are stored in two primary places: inside the fat cells deep in the abdomen, called *intra-abdominal fat,* and in the surface fat cells all over the body. While the body needs some fat stores, trouble begins when far too much energy is taken in compared to the amounts expended.

the battle ensues

When you continuously take in extra energy, more and more fatty acids are stored. As a result, the fat cells become larger and larger until a point when no more fatty acids can enter the cells. The fat cells, in an attempt to keep out any more fatty acids, develop a resistance to the insulin that is trying to force the fatty acids in. When this occurs, the fatty acids begin to build up in the

blood. To overcome the insulin resistance and move the fatty acids into the fat cells, the pancreas makes more insulin. Not to be one-upped, the fat cells further increase their insulin resistance.

As a result of this battle, you now have increased amounts of free fatty acids *and* increased levels of insulin in your bloodstream. That's bad news, because the fatty acids head back to your liver, where some are turned into triglycerides and stored in the liver,

causing a "fatty liver." The excess fatty acids also begin to irritate the liver, causing your liver enzymes to increase as well. As a response, just like your fat cells, your liver cells put up a wall of resistance to the insulin that is now trying to push the fatty acids inside. Now your liver has become resistant to insulin, and again your pancreas tries to overcome the resistance by making even more insulin. Fighting back, the liver's resistance increases, multiplying further the amounts of free fatty acids and insulin circulating in your blood.

Things go downhill from there. Remember that your body gets glucose from two sources: from the food you eat and, when you are fasting, from your liver. Insulin is responsible for controlling the glucose release from the liver. When the liver can "see" the insulin, it does not release glucose. But when insulin levels are low, your liver steps up its release of glucose.

When your liver puts up the walls of resistance to keep out the fatty acids, it can no longer "see" the insulin in the blood, so it starts to pour out extra glucose, and blood glucose levels start to rise. To combat this increase in glucose, your ever-alert pancreas pours out even more insulin, further adding to the already increasing amounts of circulating insulin.

With the liver satisfactorily keeping out the fatty acids, the fatty acids search out a new home—and they find

your muscles. Unlike your glucose-dependent brain, your muscles can use either glucose or fatty acids for energy. Because fatty acids are now very abundant and are so easy to use, your muscles switch to using fatty acids for fuel. In doing so, your muscles block the incoming glucose. They do this by building resistance to the insulin that is trying to push glucose into the muscle cells. Since your muscles are normally responsible for taking up more than 80 percent of the glucose in your blood, their switch to using fatty acids has a profound effect on your blood glucose levels. As the levels of glucose in your blood slowly start to increase above normal, you become what is called *glucose intolerant*—your tissues resist taking in glucose despite the presence of large amounts of insulin.

As blood glucose levels continue to rise, your pancreas tries in vain to lower those levels by further increasing insulin production, and your circulating insulin levels rise again. You've now entered an endless loop, with ever-increasing levels of circulating insulin, free fatty acids, and glucose, which now start to become toxic to your system.

what do you mean "toxic"?

Let's start with the fatty acids. Since the excess fatty acids cannot be made into energy by the liver, they are made into triglycerides and released into your

bloodstream. In order to make these triglycerides, your body must rob parts from other fat molecules, most specifically, from your cholesterol molecules.

One of the two main types of cholesterol molecules in your body is the *high-density lipoprotein,* or *HDL,* cholesterol. It is often called the "good" cholesterol because it removes fatty acids from your arteries so they can be eliminated from the body. The other type of cholesterol molecule is the *low-density lipoprotein,* or *LDL,* cholesterol. LDL cholesterol is often referred to as "bad" cholesterol because it tends to deposit fat in the walls of your arteries.

Unfortunately, it's the beneficial HDL molecules that take the biggest hit when the liver scavenges for parts in order to make triglycerides; the HDL level in the blood drops as a result. Parts of your LDL molecules are also used in the making of triglycerides; the effect, however, is not fewer LDL molecules but simply smaller ones. These small LDL molecules are too small to be picked out of the blood by the liver, so they don't get cleared out of the body. Instead, they continue to circulate in your blood, which allows them plenty of time to find a nice cozy weak spot on your artery walls where they can attach themselves. What you end up with, then, are high triglyceride levels, low levels of the beneficial HDL choles-terol, and a lot of small, artery-clog-ging LDL cholesterol molecules in your blood—all of which spells t-r-o-u-b-l-e for your arteries.

If that's not bad enough, you still have all that extra insulin circulating through your blood, and it's doing a number on your blood pressure. The high insulin levels caused by insulin resistance drive the blood pressure up above normal, although exactly how is unclear. The excess of insulin may result in a continuous overstimulation of the blood vessels, causing them to constrict and forcing the blood pressure above normal. In addition, the high insulin levels cause your kidneys to retain more salt, and therefore more water, which increases your blood volume; the extra blood volume, in turn, exerts greater pressure on the walls of your blood vessels.

Your high insulin levels also cause the inside lining of your blood vessels to overproduce a substance called *PAI-1* (pronounced "pie one"). PAI-1 is the main contributor to the clotting of blood. When PAI-1 levels are high, your blood clots more readily, which increases the risk of heart attack and stroke. To make matters worse, the *platelets,* tiny cells in the blood that contribute to clotting, become sticky and form clots more readily as well.

During this whole process, the ele-vated amounts of glucose in your blood start their slow, destructive process, even though the blood glucose levels may not yet have risen into the diabetic range. As discussed in the previous chapter, free radicals and AGEs begin to accumulate, affecting the tiny blood vessels of the kidneys, eyes, and feet and the large blood vessels throughout the body. Gradually, tissues throughout your body stop functioning properly.

do I have syndrome X?

Most likely, yes. More than 90 percent of people with type 2 diabetes have Syndrome X. There is no one test that confirms the diagnosis, but there are signs and laboratory tests that indicate the presence of this syndrome. If you have one or more of the following signs in addition to having type 2 dia-betes, you may have Syndrome X:

central obesity. This refers specifi-cally to the type of obesity marked by excess fat in the abdominal area as opposed to in the buttocks, hips, and thighs. This type of obesity more commonly occurs in men and in post-menopausal women.

high blood pressure (hyperten-sion). High blood pressure may be caused by the increased levels of circulating insulin, as discussed earlier. It is estimated that Syndrome X is responsible for the high blood pressure in half of all obese people.

dyslipidemia. *Dyslipidemia* means high levels of triglycerides, low levels of HDL cholesterol, and too many LDL cholesterol molecules.

angina and heart attack. In more than half the people who are seen in the hospital for angina (the chest pain caused by narrowing of the arteries leading to the heart) or a heart attack, their heart condition is caused by Syndrome X.

family history of type 2 diabetes. The majority of people with Syndrome X have a family history of type 2 diabetes. There may also be a family history of coronary artery disease.

acanthosis nigricans. *Acanthosis nigricans* is a skin condition that causes a darkening and thickening of the skin of the neck and of the body folds, such as at the armpits, in the groin area, and underneath the breasts. The elevated levels of insulin in the body stimulate the growth of skin in these areas, and the resulting skin is darker.

polycystic ovary syndrome (PCOS). This is another condition that appears to be caused by high levels of insulin. PCOS is characterized by infertility, lack of menstrual periods, and obesity. It occurs when elevated insulin levels stimulate a portion of the ovaries to overproduce male hormones, which throw off the menstrual cycle, cause acne, and increase hair growth.

what's the connection?

How is Syndrome X related to diabetes? That is a good question, and we

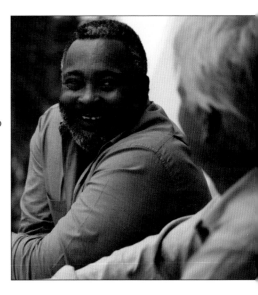

as yet do not have a complete answer. Obviously, the continued demand on the beta cells of the pancreas to produce insulin puts a strain on these cells. There may also be some toxic byproduct of insulin secretion that accumulates in the beta cells, caused by the buildup of fatty acids and rising glucose levels. These may slowly poison the beta cells. And finally, it is believed genetics may play some unknown role.

In any case, with increasing age, weight, and inactivity, the resistance to insulin increases, leading to higher and higher levels of insulin, free fatty acids, and glucose in the blood. During this "silent" period, the body is exposed to these toxins, causing high blood pressure and dyslipidemia. In 20 percent of the people who have Syndrome X, the beta cells slowly lose the ability to make insulin, and the first sign of diabetes to appear is the abnormal increase in the blood glucose level after a meal. At this stage, diabetes is usually only detected by an oral glucose tolerance test. If not diagnosed at this time, within five to ten years the elevated levels of glucose and free fatty acids lead to the further loss of insulin secretion by the pancreas. The pancreas just plain begins to poop out, overwhelmed by the demand for insulin to manage the ever-increasing levels of glucose. The increase in glucose levels now occurs even in the fasting state—upon awakening in the morning and before meals. Once the fasting glucose levels are more than 180 mg/dl, the symptoms of diabetes usually appear, sending the person to the doctor. At this point, the individual has actually had Syndrome X for more than ten years!

a one-two punch to the arteries

The combination of Syndrome X and diabetes causes the blood vessel disease atherosclerosis, also known as hardening of the arteries. Cholesterol builds up in the artery walls because there is too much LDL cholesterol in the blood and too few HDL molecules taking it away. The LDL cholesterol becomes oxidized, which makes it more irritating to the artery and often leads to a localized inflammation of the artery wall. This irritation, as well as the accumulation of fat from the LDL molecules, weakens the wall of the artery. The wall eventually cracks, causing an irregularity in the normally smooth lining of the blood vessel. The platelets and clotting factors in the blood see this wound and attach to it, which can lead to a sudden obstruction of one of the blood vessels.

If such an obstruction, or clot, occurs in the arteries feeding the heart (*coronary arteries*), it causes a sudden heart attack. If the obstruction develops more slowly, it is likely to cause angina.

A clot that occurs in the arteries to the brain, called the *cerebral arteries*, will cause either a transient ischemic attack (TIA), if the obstruction clears quickly, or a stroke. In either case, there will be sudden onset of one-sided blindness, weakness, or numbness or an inability to speak.

If the obstruction occurs in the arteries of the kidney, there will be no immediate outward symptoms. However, the blood creatinine level, which is used to gauge kidney function, will gradually worsen. This indicates that damage has been done.

If this same type of obstruction suddenly occurs in the artery to the leg, it will bring on severe leg pain, and the leg will become cold. Many times, the obstruction of the leg artery occurs slowly; this is called *claudication*. The symptoms of claudication are calf or hip pain on exertion that is relieved by rest. In a person who is not physically active, the only symptoms of claudication may be red or purple toes when the feet are dangled, loss of hair on the lower legs, thinning of the skin of the feet, or a foot ulcer.

Most people with Syndrome X and diabetes have atherosclerosis. For this reason, it is of great importance that you prevent and/or detect and treat these conditions. Very often, the symptoms of heart problems may be vague, or they may not occur at all. If you do experience any discomfort in your chest, you should contact your doctor. A screening EKG, a painless test that measures electrical signals coming from your heart, can be done to detect a problem. Although an important tool, the EKG is not very sensitive or specific, so you may need to take an exercise stress test (in which your heart function is monitored as you walk on a treadmill). Depending on your risk factors and symptoms, your doctor may also order an angiogram, a test in which dye is injected into the blood vessels to visualize any narrowing or blockage.

Likewise, if you experience any symptoms of sudden and transient vision loss in one eye or temporary weakness on one side or the other, contact your doctor at once. Your doctor can listen to the sounds of your blood flowing through the arteries in your neck (called the *carotid arteries*) to detect narrowing in these blood vessels. The doctor can then order tests of the carotid arteries to spot any obstructions.

Also, if you notice any symptoms of claudication, be sure to report them to your doctor so that the appropriate medical tests can be done to detect any blockages.

how can I treat syndrome X?

Increasing your level of activity and changing your relationship with food are a great place to start. These changes are usually inexpensive and are generally quite safe—and they are the cornerstones of treatment for both Syndrome X and diabetes. For some people, these changes are enough to decrease the levels of insulin resistance and diminish the signs of the syndrome. In addition, there are also medications available for the treatment of the various components of Syndrome X:

low-dose aspirin. A 75 to 162 mg aspirin tablet, taken daily, is moderately effective in making the platelets in your blood less "sticky," so they are less likely to attach to rough spots in your arteries. This significantly counteracts the clot-forming tendencies of Syndrome X and can reduce the risk of death from heart disease by more than one-third. If you have asthma, an aspirin allergy, or a bleeding problem, however, you should not take aspirin. In some cases, if you are taking aspirin or aspirinlike medications for chronic pain or arthritis, you may not need to take the additional low-dose aspirin for your heart. Before you consider taking a daily dose of aspirin, however, be sure to consult your doctor.

statins. Newer medications called statins have made managing dyslipidemia easy. These medications have proven themselves to be very safe and yet powerful in lowering LDL cholesterol. Common statin brands include Crestor, Lipitor, Loescol, Mevacor, Pravachol, and Zocor.

Statins all work the same way, by reducing the ability of your liver to make LDL cholesterol and by increasing your liver's take-up and destruction of the LDL cholesterol molecules in the blood. In addition, statins raise the HDL cholesterol and lower the triglyceride levels, especially when used in high doses. They are usually taken at bedtime and have few side effects. Liver irritation occurs in about 1 to 3 of every 1,000 people treated with a statin, but it usually goes away when the drug is stopped. To monitor the liver, a blood test called ALT is performed 6 to 12 weeks after starting the drug and is repeated every year. You may also experience other side effects, such as fatigue, insomnia, depression, headaches, rash, and intestinal upset, with a statin, but they are rare.

Even more rare, but potentially fatal, is *rhabdomyolysis,* which is a rapid muscle tear in your body. It is characterized by significant muscle aches and weakness all over the body and occurs more commonly when a statin is combined with certain other medications, such as erythromycin, nicotinic acid, or fibrates (Lopid or Tricor). It may also occur more often in older patients who have kidney disease. Should you experience any of these symptoms, it is very important to contact your doctor so that a simple diagnostic blood test, called a CPK, can be done.

The goal in treating cholesterol is to get the LDL cholesterol level lower than 100 mg/dl and to raise the HDL cholesterol level above 40 mg/dl in men and above 50 mg/dl in women. The goal for triglycerides is a level below 150 mg/dl. If your LDL cholesterol is more than 100 mg/dl, you should first try a statin and see what effect it has on your LDL, HDL, and triglyceride levels. If this treatment is unsuccessful and if you also have multiple risk factors for heart disease or you already have heart disease, you should discuss with your team the possibility of trying a fibrate or nicotinic acid medication.

fibrates. The fibrate medications available in the United States are Lopid and Tricor. They work directly on your liver or endothelium to reduce triglycerides and raise the HDL cholesterol level; unfortunately, they have little effect on LDL levels. Lopid appears to cause more stomach upset than does Tricor and has to be taken twice a day compared to the once-a-day dosing of Tricor. Tricor is best taken first thing in the morning. Many doctors prescribe Tricor along with a statin to get better improvements in all lipid levels, although this combination is not recommended because of the risk of muscle damage.

nicotinic acid. Also known as niacin, nicotinic acid is the best medicine for raising HDL levels. It is a vitamin, but when used in high doses, it acts as a drug. Unfortunately, such high doses of niacin also commonly cause numerous side effects, including aggravation of peptic ulcers, gout, facial flushing for a few hours after taking the medication, hives, and other skin conditions. In addition, niacin causes an *increase* in insulin resistance, which is one problem that you, as a diabetic, are trying to combat.

angiotensin converting enzyme (ACE) inhibitors. High blood pressure can be even more damaging if diabetes and Syndrome X are also present. The increased pressure in the arteries accelerates coronary and cerebrovascular disease (disease in the vessels supplying the heart and the brain, respectively) and also aggravates small-blood-vessel disease in the kidneys and eyes. So your goal is to get your blood pressure as low as possible without causing side effects, such as dizziness when you stand up. There are many new classes of medications to help you, including ACE inhibitors.

ACE inhibitors not only lower blood pressure, they also protect the lining of your blood vessels and reduce insulin resistance. In several recently reported studies, the incidence of diabetes in people who were at risk for developing it was 25 percent less in those receiving ACE inhibitors. Trials are ongoing to study whether ACE inhibitors should even be recommended as a prevention tool in those at high risk for developing diabetes.

A common side effect of ACE inhibitors is a cough. Oddly enough, the cough is a good sign. By blocking a certain chemical reaction, ACE inhibitors allow the accumulation of a chemical in the blood that is very protective to the lining of your blood vessels. The cough means that you have this protection. Rare but serious side effects of ACE inhibitors are a swelling of the mouth and tongue and an elevation in the levels of potassium and creatinine in your blood. Blood tests will need to be done before starting these medications and should be repeated after a month of treatment and then periodically thereafter. Any swelling of the mouth and tongue should be reported to your physician immediately.

There are many ACE inhibitors available, including Accupril, Altace, Capoten, Mavik, Monopril, Prinivil, and Vasotec. They are usually taken once a day and are relatively inexpensive.

angiotensin receptor blockers (ARBs). ARBs can be used in place of ACE inhibitors in people who cannot tolerate the cough caused by ACE inhibitors. ARBs block chemicals downstream from those targeted by ACE inhibitors. ARBs protect the arteries as well as ACE inhibitors do without causing a cough, but they are more expensive than ACE inhibitors. And they may still cause the other side effects that are typical of ACE inhibitors, namely, the rise in potassium and creatinine levels; therefore, follow-up blood tests are required during ARB therapy as well. A partial list of brand-name ARBs includes Avapro, Cozaar, Diovan, Micardis, and Teveten.

hydrochlorothiazides. Hydrochlorothiazides are diuretics, or "water pills." In diabetes as well as in Syndrome X, hydrochlorothiazides are used in small doses to reduce blood pressure. When given in these smaller doses, however, it does not appear that their diuretic effect is what causes a decrease in blood pressure. Rather, the small doses seem to work by relaxing the small blood vessels. In larger doses (above 12.5 mg per day), hydrochlorothiazides cause an increase in insulin resistance and a reduction in insulin secretion by the pancreas. Other side effects, again generally found in doses above 12.5 mg per day, include loss of potassium, rashes, and cramps. There are literally hundreds of brands of hydrochlorothiazides on the market, and they are very inexpensive. They are taken once a day, in the morning.

calcium channel blockers. There are several groups of compounds, called calcium channel blockers, that block the calcium channels in the muscles of the heart and blood vessels, causing the blood vessels to relax, increasing the supply of oxygen-rich blood to the heart, and decreasing the heart's workload. Of the calcium channel blockers available, the vasodilating ones (the ones that relax and widen the blood vessels) may have the fewest side effects (generally only edema and constipation) and are less expensive. They also have no negative effect on insulin resistance, which is a plus for people with diabetes. These medications include Norvasc and Plendil.

beta blockers. Beta blockers are a relatively older group of medications that have both benefits and drawbacks. The commonly used beta blockers today are Inderal, Tenormin, and Toprol. Studies have shown beta blockers to be especially effective in treating people who have coronary disease, as these drugs have been shown to reduce the chance of dying for people who have this disease. In addition, a large study conducted in England and reported in 1998 showed that Tenormin was as good as the ACE inhibitor Capoten in reducing disease of the large and small blood vessels in people with diabetes. The drawbacks to beta blockers are their side effects. They may cause nightmares, insomnia, and depression; they may block your ability to sense hypoglycemia; they may cause your hands to feel cold;

and they tend to increase insulin resistance and worsen diabetes control.

combination medications. It is also common for doctors to prescribe combinations of the above medications. For many people, successful blood pressure management occurs only with a combination of drugs. In addition, small doses of several drugs tend to cause fewer side effects than do large doses of just one. Indeed, some pharmaceutical companies have thoughtfully combined medications from different groups, such as Accupril and a hydrochlorothiazide, into one pill; the ability to take a single pill, rather than having to remember and swallow several, can in itself be a benefit.

coreg. Other drugs for treating high blood pressure have also been introduced, and some have shown great promise. One in particular, Coreg, has properties of several of the drugs discussed; it can also lower insulin resistance and reduce the oxidation of blood that occurs in Syndrome X. It can, however, cause dizziness, and it is relatively expensive.

what if my arteries are already narrowed?

Major advances have been made in unplugging heart arteries with balloons and lasers. When a sudden clot occurs, there are now powerful drugs that can dissolve the clot and keep the

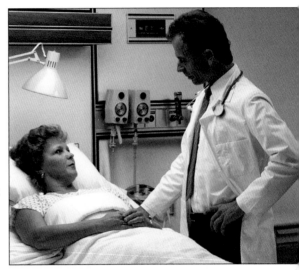

heart muscle from dying. And surgery to bypass blocked arteries is safer and less traumatic than ever. In fact, you are generally up and about within a day or two after the surgery and home before the week is out. The same is true for surgery on your carotid arteries.

If a full stroke occurs, getting to emergency care very quickly can make all the difference. Medication is now available to dissolve the clot and open the artery, although it must be given within the first few hours of the onset of the stroke. New medicines are also being developed to protect the brain or even to restore it after a stroke.

Clots in leg arteries can now often be dissolved nonsurgically, too. And newer techniques allow for surgery on smaller and smaller arteries.

Still, the best medicine is prevention. So many of the complications of diabetes and Syndrome X can be prevented by following the treatment guidelines provided by your team and maintaining control of your diabetes. Ignoring or denying the fact that you need care is the greatest risk factor of all. Fortunately, it is the one over which you have the greatest control.

children and diabetes

Diabetes is one of the most common, chronic diseases in school-age kids, affecting one of every 400 to 500 children and adolescents. Every day in America, 35 more kids are diagnosed with the disease. In the coming year, diabetes will enter the lives of nearly 13,000 more kids and their families. Because children are not simply small adults, there can be added dimensions to managing diabetes in the young.

types of diabetes in childhood

Until the last decade or so, the form of diabetes diagnosed in the majority of children was type 1, once known as juvenile diabetes. But these days, more and more children and teens are being diagnosed with type 2 diabetes, a disease traditionally seen only in adults. As evidence of this "emerging epidemic," some clinics report one-third to one-half of all new cases of childhood diabetes are now type 2. Since type 2 diabetes is more common in certain racial and ethnic groups, children who are African American, Hispanic, Latino, or Native American; who are large for their age; and who have a family history of type 2 are at especially high risk for this type.

There is a third, rare form of diabetes seen in children. It is called maturity-onset diabetes of the young (MODY), and it can occur in all ethnic groups. There are actually several varieties of MODY, all of which are caused by genetic defects that affect the insulin-producing cells. These defects are thought to be rare, and molecular diagnostic testing, currently only available in research laboratories, is required to diagnose MODY. The symptoms of MODY run the gamut from a mild increase in blood glucose to extremely high glucose levels and diabetic ketoacidosis. Treatments for MODY, therefore, range from diet and activity awareness to oral medications or insulin. Because it takes specialized testing to detect MODY, it often goes unrecognized, and most children with this form are treated as if they have either type 1 or type 2 diabetes.

managing childhood diabetes

The child who is diagnosed with type 1 diabetes is insulin dependent and requires daily injections of insulin to live. Since a child with type 1 diabetes produces little or no insulin, oral diabetes medications are not effective and are not a treatment option. Very often, shortly after starting insulin injections, the child may experience a period of reduced insulin need called the "honeymoon period." During the honeymoon period, the remaining beta cells continue to produce insulin. Insulin doses may become very low, but it is important to continue the injections during this period because even low doses of insulin appear to help prolong this "honeymoon."

A child diagnosed with type 2 diabetes is generally born into a family with a history of the disease, predisposing the child to developing it. When that predisposition is combined with environmental factors such as weight gain and inactivity, the child's blood glucose levels increase, eventually leading to diabetes. And, unfortunately, just as in adults with the disease, it is common for a child with type 2 diabetes to be insulin resistant and to have high blood pressure, high cholesterol levels, and high triglyceride

levels. So the child has an increased risk of heart disease and other diabetes complications early in life. As is the case with an adult who has the disease, the child with type 2 diabetes may need to take oral medication, insulin, or both to control the disease.

Regardless of the type of diabetes that a child has, the goal of effective diabetes management is to keep blood glucose levels as close to a "normal" range as safely possible in order to reduce the long- and short-term complications of diabetes and to promote normal growth and development. The target blood glucose range must be determined individually for each child.

children are not small adults

Managing diabetes takes commitment and effort regardless of when it develops. But diabetes presents unique issues for children and teens with the disease. For example, the simple pleasures of childhood, such as going to birthday parties, basketball games, or sleepovers, need careful planning for the child with diabetes.

Every day, the child with diabetes may need to take insulin or oral medication. The child's blood glucose level will have to be checked several times a day, and food intake and activity will have to be accounted for. Depending on the child's age, these are burdens assumed by the caregiver alone, shared between

Do as I do

One of the best ways to help a child who has, or is at risk for developing, type 2 diabetes is to make lifestyle improvement a family affair.

Set a good example and involve everyone. Learn together about smarter eating and activity choices. Then explore them together.

Tackle the produce section at the grocery or farmers market. Give everyone a chance to pick a new fruit or vegetable for the whole family to try. Experiment with different colors, flavors, and textures. Explore some fresh herbs and spices in place of added salt and fat.

Next, get active together. Try doing some chores by hand or errands on foot. For fun, go on family bike rides or family walks. Spend a day at a local park or museum. You might even consider taking an activity-based family vacation. Go ahead, get creative. Then, get going!

an older child and the caregiver, or assumed completely by the teenager.

For the parent or other caregiver, who is essentially playing the role of the child's pancreas, the sheer responsibility can be daunting; it is a job that is impossible to do perfectly. And it is easy for the caregiver to become overwhelmed by the daily demands of determining exact insulin amounts, anticipating the child's carbohydrate intake and activity levels, and preventing both hypoglycemia (which, if it is not treated, can cause brain damage) and high blood sugar levels (which, if poorly controlled, can increase the long-term complications). What's more, the stress of caring for a child with diabetes can aggravate any psychological, social, or financial problems that the family may already be experiencing. Because the diagnosis of diabetes changes a family and its dynamics forever, seeking and getting social and psychological support is essential for the well-being of all the family members.

As a child grows older and the daily responsibility of diabetes management shifts, the stress shifts as well. These years of transition, as the older child gradually learns self-management skills and develops personal judgment, are

not often easy on the child or the family. The typical confusion and frustration that come with being a teenager can be aggravated by the stress of managing diabetes, even causing emotional and behavioral problems. Learning to cope with diabetes in adolescence is a big job, and reaching out to health professionals for additional support may help the teenager, the parents, and other family members.

The child's diabetes care team is an important resource and can often suggest care and treatment options that can help ease some of the difficulties. For example, a child who requires insulin daily may benefit from the use of an insulin pump (see the chapter Using Insulin). The pump not only improves control but helps restore some flexibility and spontaneity to the family's lifestyle and schedule. With the pump, gone are the schedules of meals, snacks, and shots; there is also less risk of hypoglycemia. In addition, using the pump allows significantly more freedom in food choices and amounts.

Because so much of a child's life is spent in the classroom, it's also important to bring teachers and school officials into the loop as an added safety net. There are now laws to ensure that children with diabetes are treated fairly at school and that the child's medical needs are met. These laws apply to all public schools and most private schools and day care centers. All schools must

Type of diabetes	WHICH RELATIVE HAS DIABETES?	YOUR CHANCE OF GETTING DIABETES
Type 1	Your brother, sister, son, or daughter	10%
Type 1	Your mother	4%
Type 1	Your father	10%
Type 2	Your brother or sister	25%
Type 2	Your mother or father	12%
Type 2	Your mother and father	50%
Type 2	Your identical twin	90%

have a written plan for the child with diabetes. It must clearly state when the child needs to check blood sugar and take insulin, the timing of meals and snacks, the symptoms and treatment of high and low blood sugar, and the phone numbers for parents and other emergency contacts.

Yet another resource that can help ease the burden for the child and provide a break for the caregiver are the various camps for children with diabetes. Camp provides a great opportunity for children and teenagers who have diabetes to get to know others who face the same challenges and to have fun in a safe environment while learning useful coping skills. An excellent resource for exploring diabetes camps in your area can be found at www.childrenwithdiabetes.com/camps.

it's nature *and* nurture: they both play a role

For the average American, the chance of developing type 1 diabetes by age 70 is 1 in 100 (1 percent), while the risk of type 2 is 1 in 9 (11 percent). However, having a family member with the disease changes these odds, especially for type 2 diabetes (see the chart above). Type 2 seems to run in families more often than does type 1.

While type 2 has a strong genetic link, it is heavily influenced by lifestyle. In other words, a child who doesn't have a family history of type 2 but who lives in an environment of inactivity and free-flowing calories can develop type 2 diabetes quite easily. Conversely—and fortunately—even a family history of diabetes doesn't condemn a child to developing type 2 if the child learns healthy diet and exercise habits.

use your diabetes tool kit

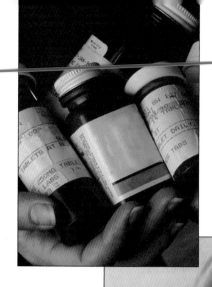

A diagnosis of diabetes can be disheartening, but there is plenty of good news. These days, you have a well-stocked kit of diabetes tools available to help you keep your blood sugar under tight control and ward off the frightening complications associated with diabetes. You simply need to understand how to apply them to your best advantage and to commit yourself to using them faithfully. You'll learn about these tools— blood sugar monitoring, HbA1c testing, adjusting your diet and physical activity, using pills and insulin, and preparing for low blood sugar events—as well as how you and your diabetes care team can get the most from them, here in this section.

monitoring your glucose

To achieve glucose levels that are as close to normal as possible, you need to monitor them regularly. Today, the meters available for glucose testing are small, convenient, and relatively easy to use, making monitoring an easier and more effective part of your diabetes care. What's more, new testing methods on the horizon may one day make testing automatic and painless.

to master, you must monitor

Blood glucose monitoring is a vital part of the diabetes management process, and frequent self-monitoring is the key to successful diabetes care. By testing your glucose, you get a precise measurement of what your blood glucose level is at the time of the test so you can adjust your food, medication, or activity level accordingly and with confidence. It means far greater freedom to participate in any activities you choose and, therefore, far greater control over your life. The blood glucose values are like clues in a mystery novel. The more clues you have, the greater your understanding of the mystery. Of course, the opposite can be true as well. The less you test, the fewer clues you have and the more your diabetes remains a mystery to both you and your diabetes care team.

Checking your blood glucose level is essential in managing your diabetes because it is a critical factor in making treatment decisions to prevent the potentially devastating effects of diabetes. Research has shown that the higher blood glucose is allowed to be over time, the greater the possibility of problems and serious complications that affect many systems of the body. A national study, the Diabetes Control and Complications Trial, has shown that tightly controlling blood glucose levels can prevent, reduce, or even reverse some of the long-term complications and problems associated with diabetes. It was this study that showed that by maintaining your blood glucose level as close to normal as possible, you may reduce your risk of complications involving your eyes, kidneys, and nervous system by up to 60 percent.

This level of tight glucose control depends on frequent monitoring. Even for the person whose daily routine rarely changes, all kinds of things, such as stress, illness, unanticipated activity, alcohol, or medications, can throw off the balanced routine, resulting in unpleasant and sometimes dangerous glucose fluctuations.

Testing your blood glucose on a regular basis allows you to know the ongoing status of your diabetes and will help you learn more about your diabetes and your body. Testing multiple times each day will give you even more information. Such frequent testing helps you understand blood glucose patterns that occur when you eat certain foods and take specific medication doses and how these are connected to your level of activity and stressors at home or work. Frequent testing also ensures that you can respond quickly to high or low blood glucose with appropriate intervention.

Your monitor records how your personal glucose levels change in response to ordinary events, such as eating, menstruation, stress, and activity. Then, working together with your diabetes care team and through careful trial and error, you can find out what works best for you—food, exercise, medications, or insulin—to keep your levels as close to normal as possible.

If you choose not to test your blood glucose levels, you cannot know whether your diabetes is really controlled. You never learn the relationship between what and how much you eat and your blood glucose levels. The lows that occur, say, after activity will remain a mystery, as will the high blood glucose levels that may be occurring each morning. Only with frequent glucose testing can you monitor your levels and be assured that they are within the normal range. When done properly, and with support and education from your diabetes care team, glucose testing can allow *you* to modify the type of food you eat, vary the amount and time you exercise, and adjust your medications.

what meter is best for me?

Blood glucose monitoring systems are easier, faster, and more accurate than ever. Many

Why would I want to test my blood glucose?

- To identify patterns in my blood glucose control
- To lead a more flexible life
- To reduce the risk of long-term diabetes complications
- To understand the impact of food, activity, and medications on my blood glucose
- To quickly identify either a high or low glucose level and treat the problem appropriately
- To figure out what may be causing my high or low blood glucose levels
- So my diabetes care team has to do less guessing when establishing a treatment plan for me
- To determine the effectiveness of my current diabetes treatment plan and identify when changes are needed
- To evaluate changes in my diabetes treatment plan and see if my glucose levels improve
- Because numbers are information, and with information I can better manage my disease
- To learn, with the help of my team, how to modify my food intake, level of activity, and medications and still maintain healthy glucose levels
- Because testing allows me to reach a level of freedom, security, and control that would otherwise be impossible
- To feel good
- To live healthy, well, and free from the complications of diabetes

meters give test results in seconds, and most will store results for later recall. Meters include many features designed specifically to make self-monitoring convenient. Many operate on batteries, are small enough to fit in a purse or shirt pocket, and can be used almost anywhere. Some have an electronic memory, and more-advanced models even contain built-in modems for transmitting the test results to your physician. With so many options available, you should look at several models and discuss their advantages and disadvantages with your diabetes care team to see which model best suits your needs.

The meters that are currently available use one of two methods for measuring blood glucose. The *reflectance photometers* measure light reflected from a test strip after it has undergone a chemical reaction. Photometric meters have been around the longest and have proven to be reliable and accurate. They use a light source with filters and a lens to detect a color change on the strip caused by glucose in the blood. The *electrochemical meters* measure the electric current produced by the blood resting on the tip of the test strip. Electrochemical meters use the newest technology currently available. Glucose in the blood causes a reaction on the test strip that produces a tiny electric current, and the meter detects and "reads" the current. Regardless of their type, all meters on the U.S. market have been tested for accuracy and approved for home use by the U.S. Food and Drug Administration (FDA).

In addition to the two methods of measuring blood glucose, meters are also calibrated in one of two ways. Your test results are either reported as a *whole-blood reading* or are *plasma calibrated*. Whole-blood meters measure the glucose present in a drop of whole blood. Plasma-calibrated meters measure the glucose present in a drop of whole blood but then automatically add 12 percent to the measured value. This plasma-calibrated value is equal to the reading that a laboratory might obtain, since all laboratory equipment is set up to measure the glucose that is present in a plasma sample of blood. (A plasma sample is the portion of the blood that remains once the red blood cells are removed.) One type of reading is no better than the other. They both measure your blood glucose. You just need to know how your meter is calibrated so you and your team can set appropriate goals and you can correctly determine the accuracy of your meter when comparing it to a laboratory test result.

When narrowing your choice of meters, and in order to get the most benefit from your monitoring, you should pick the meter that you find easiest to use and maintain properly. This is crucial: You have to be able to perform the procedure properly to get reliable and accurate results. And you have to find a meter easy enough for you to use and maintain, or you'll be tempted to skip regular testing.

REQUIRED?		FEATURES TO CONSIDER WHEN CHOOSING A METER
YES	NO	Does the speed of testing make a difference? *(Meters can take anywhere from 6 seconds to 2 minutes to provide glucose results.)*
YES	NO	Do you want a meter that "beeps" to prompt you?
YES	NO	Do you want a silent meter?
YES	NO	Is the meter simple to use? Are there a lot of complicated steps required to operate the meter each time you need to check your glucose level?
YES	NO	Do you prefer individually wrapped test strips? *(Some people find the foil-wrapped strips difficult to open, but such strips are less prone to spoilage if you use the meter in an area of high humidity.)*
YES	NO	Is the calibration test easy to perform?
YES	NO	Does the meter need to be cleaned? If so, is it an easy procedure?
YES	NO	Do you need a meter with a memory?
YES	NO	Do you want the meter memory to give you the date and time of the glucose test in addition to the test result?
YES	NO	Do you want the meter memory to hold more than ten glucose tests?
YES	NO	Do you want a meter that can record your insulin dose and other information as well?
YES	NO	Do you want a meter that can download its memory to a computer?
YES	NO	If your diabetes care team downloads your meter information at your visits, is the meter compatible with your team's system?
YES	NO	Will you be using the meter at high altitudes or in extreme temperatures? If so, are you able to use the meter under such varying conditions?
YES	NO	Do you have trouble getting a blood sample from your fingers? If so, does this meter require a very small sample of blood?
YES	NO	Would you prefer to use a test site other than your fingers, such as your arms or legs, to get a blood sample? If so, does this meter allow for it?
YES	NO	If you pay for your test strips yourself, are they affordable? *(This will be your largest expense over the long haul. The difference between meter costs is small compared to the ongoing cost of the test strips.)*
YES	NO	If the meter requires batteries, are the batteries easy to replace and convenient to find? *(Some meter companies will give you a new meter when the batteries are low.)*
YES	NO	Do you want a plasma-calibrated meter?

Meters themselves are usually relatively inexpensive. Many machines are actually available for free at pharmacies and clinics through special offers from manufacturers. Some manufacturers give you a meter free with the purchase of test strips. Most manufacturers of meters offer mail-in rebates after you buy the meter and trade-in rebates if you mail them back your old meter. This way, if you don't like your original purchase, you can always trade it in for another at little or no cost. It is important to keep in mind, however, that you should never trade in your current meter based solely on the fact that the new one is free. Check and see if the new, free meter has all the features you feel are important, and also check with your diabetes care team to see if the trade would be a "good deal" for you.

If you have insurance, check with your provider regarding the coverage of diabetes supplies and which meters and supplies, if specified, are covered. If you have Medicare, regulations in effect since July 1998 specify that Medicare will cover the costs of blood testing supplies for people with diabetes. Check with your local Medicare provider for details.

There are currently some 30 different meters available in the United States alone. Your choice of meter will depend, at least in part, on the individual features of the meters. Use the checklist on page 49 to help determine which features you prefer and/or require in your meter.

Chapters could be devoted to all the meter systems available on the market today. In addition, you could spend days, even weeks, traveling from pharmacy to pharmacy to see demonstrations of all the different meters. In general, no single store will have every meter available for you to evaluate.

Keeping all of this in mind, you might find it easiest to begin your search via the Internet or with a good, nonbiased reference guide. One of the best references is the buyer's guide published yearly in the December issue of the American Diabetes Association's *Diabetes Forecast* magazine. This buyer's guide can also be found on the Diabetes Association's Web site at www.diabetes.org/diabetesforecast. All of the information is voluntarily supplied by the various product manufacturers. The American Diabetes Association does not review, endorse, or compare products but rather presents information about each category of products from those manufacturers who choose to provide it.

when should I test?

A study published in the *British Journal of Medicine* showed that frequent blood glucose testing played a greater role in lowering blood glucose levels than did any medication, diet, or exercise plan available to treat diabetes. It showed that the more often a person tested their blood glucose levels in a day, the better their blood glucose control overall. And further research has shown that the better the glucose control overall, the lower the risk of long-term complications of diabetes.

So, the best time to test is . . . as often as possible! Most people find that, generally, the best times to check blood glucose levels are just prior to meals and before crawling into bed. You may also find it extremely helpful to test one to two hours after you eat to see the effect of food on your glucose levels. By using your meter to check your blood glucose level at different times of the day, you begin collecting valuable information and get a good idea of how well your treatment program is working.

what should my numbers be?

Your personal blood glucose goals will depend on your age, the type of diabetes you have and how long you've had it, any other health conditions you suffer from, your lifestyle, and your desired level of control. You should check with your diabetes care team to determine the best range of blood glucose levels for you. The American Diabetes Association (ADA) has set as the standard of care for people with diabetes:

• before-meal goals of 90–130 mg/dl

• less than 180 mg/dl at any time after a meal

Remember, when setting your blood glucose goals with your team, you need to take into account the type of meter you are using—whether it's a plasma-calibrated or whole-blood meter. The standards set by the ADA are for plasma-calibrated meters. If you are using a whole-blood meter, you and your team need to subtract 12 percent from the stated goals. Always be sure to inform your diabetes care team every time you change meters to determine if any changes are needed in your treatment program or in your target blood glucose ranges. In addition, if you change meter types or begin using more than one type of meter to do your testing, be sure you know how each meter is calibrated.

Finally, a word of caution. If your doctor does not ask you to do glucose testing or discourages the frequency of your testing, beware. You are not receiving the standard of care as recommended by the American Diabetes Association and the American Association of Diabetes Educators.

am I doing this right?

Obtaining a drop of blood is sometimes the most difficult part of blood glucose testing. Many meter manufacturers now provide lancing devices that can be adjusted to varying depths, depending on individual need, which

When to test more often

There are certain times when you may want to increase the frequency of your testing, for example:
• If you begin to feel "odd" or ill
• Before and after exercise
• One, two, and three hours after eating when you want to know how a specific food affects your glucose levels
• When you start a new medication (especially a steroid), so you can closely monitor its effect
• During periods of stress, illness, or surgery
• If you become pregnant
• When you suspect your blood glucose level is high or low
• Any time there are changes to your daily routine or treatment program, such as in medication dose, meal plan, or activity level

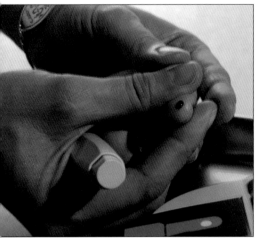

helps reduce the pain of testing and improves the chances of obtaining an adequate sample.

Immediately before each test, make sure your hands are clean and free from anything that could influence your reading. When you wash your hands, use warm water. After drying, shake your hands below your waist and then squeeze, or milk, your test finger a few times before you lance a site. Make sure you use a new lancet before each test to ensure that it is clean and sharp. Place the lancet lightly against your finger on the side of the pad, where there are fewer nerve endings, then push the lancet in to obtain your blood sample.

If you have ongoing problems obtaining an adequate sample to perform the test, talk with your diabetes care team for suggestions. You may also want to explore using one of the alternate-site meters that allow you to obtain a blood sample from your arms or legs.

As previously discussed, testing is a vital part of managing your diabetes. However, appropriate decisions regarding changes in your medications, eating, and level of activity can be made only if the results of your blood tests are accurate. According to an FDA-sponsored study, the main factors behind inaccurate readings appear to be inadequate training in the use of meters and a misunderstanding of the manufacturer's instructions, leading to errors in the operation of the meter.

The most common errors that were found among meter-users were:
- failure to follow the manufacturer's instructions
- inadequate amount and improper placement of blood on the test strip
- failure to calibrate the meter
- lack of proper cleaning of the device
- the use of outdated test strips

Based on the FDA study, suggestions were made for reducing these errors. It was recommended that you:
- obtain professional training and guidance for the use of your particular meter
- make sure you are using fresh strips and supplies
- clean your meter frequently (or use a meter that does not require cleaning)
- check your testing technique routinely with a professional
- follow the manufacturer's meter instructions carefully

If you faithfully follow these suggestions but suspect that your meter values are incorrect, reread the manufacturer's instructions. Then check the calibration of the meter, and run a control test using the solution provided by the meter company. Repeat your blood glucose test again. If the meter's results still don't seem right, contact your diabetes care team or call the meter manufacturer's 800 number, which is usually located on the back of the meter.

What if your meter reading doesn't match the laboratory's results for the same blood sample? Your meter reading is considered accurate if its results fall within 20 percent, plus or minus, of the laboratory results after any necessary calibration conversions are made.

Remember that blood glucose meters and laboratory equipment measure glucose in different ways. Lab equipment uses only the plasma portion of blood to measure blood glucose, which means that the red blood cells are removed before glucose is measured. All blood glucose meters, on the other hand, measure the glucose level in whole blood, which is 12 percent lower. If you use a plasma-calibrated meter, you don't have to be concerned about that 12 percent difference, because your meter automatically makes that adjustment. Your results can be compared directly with those from the lab. And if they fall within 20 percent of each other, your testing is on target.

If, however, you use a noncalibrated whole-blood meter, you will need to do a mathematical conversion on the lab results in order to compare them to your own results. To do this, simply divide the lab results by 1.12. If your

EXAMPLE OF CALCULATION TO FIGURE ACCEPTABLE RANGE WHEN COMPARING YOUR METER RESULT TO A LAB RESULT OF **231**			
PLASMA-CALIBRATED METER		**WHOLE-BLOOD METER**	
$231 \times .20 = 46$	Variance	$231 \div 1.12 = 206$	Converted Result
$231 + 46 = 277$	Acceptable High	$206 \times .20 = 41$	Variance
$231 - 46 = 185$	Acceptable Low	$206 + 41 = 247$	Acceptable High
Acceptable Meter Range = 185 – 277		$206 - 41 = 165$	Acceptable Low
Which is ±20% of 231		Acceptable Meter Range = 165 – 247	
		Which is ±20% of 206	

meter results fall within plus or minus 20 percent of the converted number, your testing is on target.

If, despite rechecking your calculations, the lab results and your meter results aren't close enough, report this to your diabetes care team.

what do I do with the numbers?

If you are putting in the time, money, and effort to test your blood glucose levels regularly, then you sure want something to come of your efforts. Try as you might, you will never be able to say for certain that you have complete control of your blood glucose levels. You will not be able to wake up one morning and confidently state that "All of my glucose levels will be under 140 today." You can, however, use the numbers that you get to help you confidently manage your diabetes.

To get the most out of your testing, you need a few pieces of information. First, make sure you know the correct way to perform a test. Next, know your target glucose levels, and figure out the best times to test your levels to give yourself and your team the most information. Finally, record your tests, even if your meter has a memory and you or your team can download the numbers from your meter.

When you keep a written record, not only do you have the time, date, and glucose levels that the meter records, but you are also able to record essential, and sometimes critical, information. Record the type and dose of each diabetes medicine you take and the time you take it. (Do not fill out your record book ahead of time; your dose may change at some point or you may forget to take a dose. You want the record to accurately reflect what is

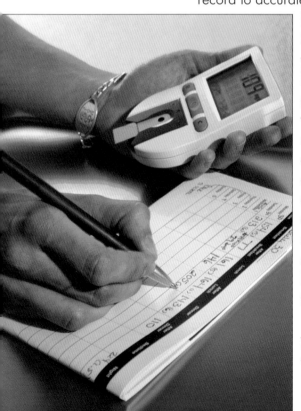

happening to you.) Record changes in your routine that may be affecting your glucose levels. You will want to note any unusual events such as changes in mealtimes or the amount of food eaten, changes in activity, illness, or unusual stress. Also be sure to record any hypoglycemic events that occur.

With such detail, you and your team can identify glucose

patterns and determine what causes your blood glucose fluctuations. You'll have enough information to manage your diabetes and develop a plan to get your blood glucose levels into your target range.

Keeping this written record is vital. You and your diabetes care team can use this information to make safe adjustments to your diet, level of activity, insulin, or oral medications. A well-kept record can help you and your team see patterns in your level of control. Always have your professionals "think out loud" when they make changes in your treatment plan. Ask them what they saw in your record of glucose levels to prompt a change. How do they think the change will affect your future values? Make sure you understand their thinking and logic. In this way, with time and practice, you may be able to do the same type of management.

meter choices today and tomorrow

When it comes to blood glucose monitoring, the real excitement and anticipation centers around the coming of meters that measure blood glucose levels without needing a skin puncture to get a blood sample for each reading. Fortunately, the pipeline is full of breakthrough technologies that will revolutionize the monitoring of blood glucose and, as a result, the care of diabetes. A couple of early innovators in this area are already breaking out of the gate.

In 1999, the FDA granted approval to Medtronic MiniMed for their continuous glucose monitoring system, which automatically monitors the glucose level in the patient with diabetes. It requires that a sensor be implanted just under the skin on the patient's abdomen for up to three days. It records glucose levels every five to six minutes during that time. The record is then downloaded in the doctor's office, and from the resultant printouts, the doctor can analyze the glucose fluctuations that occurred during the three days and make recommendations for improving the patient's pattern of eating, medication administration, and activity level to improve blood glucose control. At present, the sensor does not provide on-demand blood glucose readings; the results must be downloaded. And it is currently available only for use under a doctor's care to monitor the patient's glucose levels over a 48- to 72-hour period.

Further advancements were made in February 2004, when the Guardian system from Medtronic MiniMed was approved by the FDA for patient use. The Guardian is an expanded version of the continuous glucose monitoring system, designed to protect the patient

with diabetes by alerting them to potentially dangerous fluctuations in blood glucose levels. By sounding an alarm when glucose levels become too high or too low, the system warns the patient to take action to normalize their blood sugar, which can result in improved health and quality of life. Like the system available in the physician's office, the monitor can be downloaded to a computer for additional trend analysis.

Another breakthrough device, the GlucoWatch Biographer, received FDA approval for patient home use in March 2001. While the watchlike device measures and displays glucose readings up to every ten minutes, it is intended as a supplement to, not a replacement for, your blood glucose meter. The device uses a process that involves applying a small electric current to the skin—using a AAA battery—whenever glucose levels are to be measured. As with the Guardian, you can set personal glucose alert levels so that an alarm sounds if readings are too high or too low.

The race is on, and while these are the first competitors out of the gates, there are more than a dozen companies with products soon to hit the market. Such devices promise to be the biggest step forward in diabetes self-management in 30 years.

HbA1c: looking back to move forward

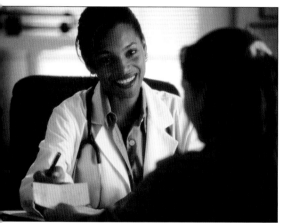

The blood glucose testing you do at home provides incredibly valuable information about your glucose levels. Each test you perform tells you what your glucose level is at that particular point in time, so that you can take steps immediately to bring a high or low level back under control. But there is yet another essential tool that you and your doctor can use to monitor your glucose levels and make decisions about your diabetes treatment. It's a laboratory test called the *glycohemoglobin* (or *HbA1c*) *test,* and it can help you and your doctor evaluate your level of glucose control over the previous several weeks. Testing for glycohemoglobin does not replace the blood glucose testing you do at home. Rather, it adds to the information you and your doctor can use to manage your diabetes.

what is glycohemoglobin?

Inside your red blood cells is a protein called *hemoglobin* that is responsible for carrying oxygen from your lungs to all the tissues in your body. Glucose that's circulating in your blood can attach to, or *glycate,* the hemoglobin inside the red blood cell, forming *glycohemoglobin.* Once the glucose attaches to the hemoglobin, it stays there as long as the red blood cell lives, which is generally about two to three months. Red blood cells don't turn over, or die, all at once (otherwise, you'd be without oxygen until they could be replaced). Old ones are constantly dying, and new ones are constantly being made. You might say that, at any one time, your red blood cells are a mix of the very old, the middle aged, and the quite young, with more of them being on the younger side of their lives.

Normally, in someone who does not have diabetes, about 4 to 6 percent of the hemoglobin in their blood is coated in glucose. In the person with diabetes, who has blood glucose levels that are higher than normal, more glucose attaches to the hemoglobin molecules. For the person with diabetes, usually anywhere from less than 6 percent to more than 20 percent of their hemoglobin molecules are coated in glucose. The glycohemoglobin, or HbA1c, blood test measures this percentage. And because some of the hemoglobin molecules are older and some newer, the test results provide a backward glance at the average glucose levels over the past two to three months. Looking at these numbers can help you and your doctor evaluate how well your current diabetes therapy is working and whether any adjustments need to be made to improve your blood glucose control.

It is recommended that a person who has diabetes have an HbA1c test at least twice a year. More frequent glycohemoglobin testing is warranted in certain situations, such as when a new medication or treatment regimen is being tried or when blood glucose goals simply aren't being met.

Unfortunately, unlike blood cholesterol testing or blood pressure measurement, there is no one standard value, no consistently defined "healthy range" used by every single laboratory that performs HbA1c testing. As a result, it can be difficult to compare results from different laboratories and hard to communicate guidelines to the public as well as to professionals.

There is hope that one day all laboratories will use a standard scale for HbA1c measurement. And there has been some progress in that direction. Ever since a study called the Diabetes Control and Complications Trial (DCCT) showed the benefits of HbA1c measurements in helping to stave off diabetes complications, many laboratories have started using testing methods that bring their values in line with the ranges used in the DCCT. Furthermore, the HbA1c recommendations from the American Diabetes Association apply only to laboratories that use testing methods that are "certified as traceable" to the DCCT trial method.

For now, however, you and your doctor need to find out what the "normal range" values are at the laboratory you use in order to interpret your results properly and use them to evaluate your glucose control. Be sure to make a note of this range for your own future reference.

what does an HbA1c number mean?

In general, when evaluating an HbA1c test, each percent increase in the hemoglobin A1c reflects an increase in average blood glucose of 35 mg/dl. So, if an HbA1c of 6 percent is equal to an average blood glucose level of 135 mg/dl, then 7 percent would be

Why is it called HbA1c?

The term glycohemoglobin actually refers to a family of glucose-coated hemoglobin molecules. One of these, *hemoglobin A1c,* or simply *HbA1c,* is considered the most stable member when it comes to long-term glucose measurement. In addition, because of its stability, the HbA1c value is not affected by a meal eaten right before the test, so there's no need to fast before you give blood for the test. Because of these factors, when you are having a glycohemoglobin test, it's most likely your HbA1c that is actually being measured.

equal to 170 mg/dl, 8 percent would equal 205 mg/dl, and so on. The American Diabetes Association recommends that the hemoglobin A1c goal be less than 7 percent for people with diabetes. (Again, these recommended values apply to test results performed using a testing method certified as traceable to the Diabetes Control and Complications Trial method.) Most studies, however, have shown that only when the hemoglobin A1c is less than 6 percent is there no increase in diabetes complications.

why bother with home blood tests?

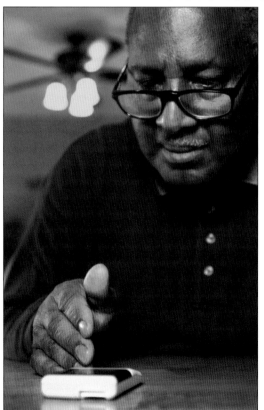

As previously mentioned, HbA1c testing is not a substitute for your own daily blood glucose monitoring. The HbA1c measures only the *average* glucose level over the past two to three months. It can provide you with an overall picture of how well you have been controlling your blood glucose over time, whether your current treatment plan is helping to maintain or improve your control, and whether a shift in your plan is needed. The HbA1c can't, however, tell you what your blood glucose level is at any one point in time; that's why home blood glucose testing is so important.

The blood glucose monitoring you do at home gives you specific information about your glucose level at the time of the test. It allows you to take immediate action to keep your blood glucose from going way too high or way too low. Based on the reading, you may decide that you need a snack, for example, or more insulin. It's the overall effectiveness of these individual day-to-day decisions, which you make based on your daily blood testing, that is reflected in your HbA1c.

The two types of testing—at-home blood tests and HbA1c tests—also serve as cross-checks for one another. For example, say your record of blood glucose tests for the past couple of months indicates your levels have been in a range that reflects excellent control of diabetes. But the HbA1c test results you just received suggest a much poorer level of control over that same time period. It's possible that something went wrong with the HbA1c test. But it is also possible that you are not doing the home blood tests properly or often enough or that your meter is not providing accurate results. Without feedback from both of these tests, you might never have known there was something wrong. Getting to the bottom of these contradictory results may help you and your doctor identify a problem in your current treatment plan. Once it's identified, you and your diabetes care team can take steps to remedy the problem and improve your control.

If your HbA1c value does not seem to agree with the average of the values recorded by your blood glucose meter (some meters provide you with an average of your readings over a specified period of time; otherwise, you can simply add up all the readings as you've recorded them in your log and divide that by the total number of entries to get your average), you should ask yourself the following questions:

- Am I testing frequently enough? Checking four times a day and occasionally one hour after meals should indicate your average value.

- Have I been testing long enough? You need to take the average of at least six-weeks' worth of blood glucose readings to get a valid comparison to the HbA1c.

- Is my meter accurate? Using a single blood sample, compare the readings from your meter against readings from your doctor's meter or from the lab (see the chapter Monitoring Your Glucose for more information on this procedure).

- Do I have a medical condition that may be affecting the accuracy of my HbA1c tests? There are some instances in which HbA1c testing can give you a false impression. When certain conditions are present, for example, your hemoglobin molecules can have a shorter than normal life span, resulting in artificially low HbA1c values. Such conditions include anemia caused by blood loss, pregnancy, renal (kidney) disease, and vitamin deficiencies. Rarely, the HbA1c value can be artificially high as a result of abnormalities in the hemoglobin itself; in such cases, HbA1c values can even reach levels above 50 percent.

If you've been testing long enough, if your meter's readings appear to be accurate, and if conditions that affect hemoglobin have been ruled out as possible factors, ask your doctor to redo your HbA1c test. If there is still a discrepancy, you will need to work with your diabetes care team to determine and correct the problem.

Relationship between HbA1c and average blood glucose

Your hemoglobin A1c value (HbA1c) is equal to an average blood glucose over the last two to three months. The American Diabetes Association recommends that your HbA1c value be less than 7 percent to reduce your long-term complications of diabetes. A level that is below 6 percent is an even better target to aim for.

Another formula you can use to determine your exact blood glucose average is:

$$(HbA1c \times 35) - 75 = \text{Average Blood Glucose}$$

HbA1c %	AVERAGE BLOOD GLUCOSE (MG/DL)
13.0%	380
12.0%	345
11.0%	310
10.0%	275
9.0%	240
8.0%	205
7.0%	170
6.0%	135
5.0%	100

eating for better control

Eating is essential to life, but we eat for many reasons: out of hunger or habit, for pleasure, even as a way of dealing with emotions. A diagnosis of diabetes can make the simple act of eating seem overwhelmingly complicated. With education and experimentation, however, you can turn eating into a powerful diabetes management tool.

there is no diabetes diet anymore

When you learned you had diabetes, you may have assumed you'd have to go on a special, restrictive diet. Perhaps you'd heard of people with diabetes who had to give up every food they enjoyed or who stopped going to certain events or restaurants because there was nothing they could eat there. Well, cheer up. You don't need to follow a "diabetic diet" anymore.

A *diet* implies that you need to eat sparingly or according to strict prescribed rules. Diets also have a nasty habit of prohibiting rich, high-calorie, mouthwatering foods. Research shows that dieters often report overwhelming desires for the foods they're *not* supposed to eat on a diet and that they often give in to those cravings. Once they give in, they frequently over-indulge. This diet/binge cycle is very common in those who frequently go on weight-loss diets. It leads not only to failed weight-loss attempts but to weight regain, yo-yo dieting, feelings of guilt, and constant food cravings.

The traditional diabetic diet is really no different than traditional weight-loss diets; indeed, it prescribes even greater food restrictions and pretty much dictates what foods are and are not allowed. Likewise, studies have shown that those following a traditional diabetic diet are no different than other dieters—they, too, eventually give in to their desires and binge on "forbidden foods." For the person with diabetes, falling off the traditional diabetes diet wagon leads not only to weight regain, guilt, and constant cravings but to something potentially more dangerous—poor diabetes control.

The actual problem with diets in general—and the source of the on-going diet/binge cycle and constant food cravings—is that dieting is based on four flawed assumptions:

1. The first flawed assumption is that eating is always done in a continuous state of awareness. For some

people, however, eating comes close to being on the same level of consciousness as breathing. Have you ever found that you've polished off a whole box of crackers or some other snack and don't even remember taking the first bite? Somehow eating, like breathing, just happened without any thought. That's not to say that for periods of time a person can't focus intently on a diet, following every rule and detail. It's just that, in time, the spell will be broken and the person will drift back to old eating habits.

2. A diet presumes that we eat only to provide our bodies with fuel. But many people have strong expectations to have certain foods at certain times and places. Diets rarely take into consideration birthday or holiday celebrations, complete with traditional foods and cultural associations. Nor do they take into account Dad's classic Sunday brunch extravaganza or Grandma's jar full of buttery homemade cookies. Only certain foods and food combinations will do at these times, otherwise it's just not the same.

3. Diets work on the belief that all of your emotional needs are met. Cravings for food and the need to eat may be responses to stresses in your life that need to be addressed. A diet discounts the need for comfort foods that calm and that are eaten in an attempt to soothe away life's troubles and turmoil. These foods have pleasurable tastes and textures and are used as rewards or to provide solace, a practice commonly begun in childhood and continued throughout life.

4. Diets operate on the idea that demand should equal supply. In other words, when a diet restricts certain foods, your desire or demand for them should not increase. However, just the opposite tends to be true. The deprivation of dieting sets you up to long for, think about, and plan your days around foods that you *cannot* or *should not* eat. It becomes a simple case of wanting what you can't have.

It's foolish and, in the end, self-defeating to deny the associations we have with food and the emotions certain foods evoke. Attempting to ignore these influences, which is what we try to do anytime we "go on a diet," sets us up for disordered eating behaviors, such as bingeing and overeating. By trying to totally avoid certain foods, people instead tend to overconsume them in the end. For you, the person with diabetes, this can lead to additional problems. You may skip your glucose testing or not record results—you may even cancel medical appointments—because you figure you've "blown" your diet and testing your blood sugar would just remind you of your failure.

Rather than a restrictive diet, what you need is knowledge and information. You need to understand how food fuels and affects your body, especially your glucose levels, and then use that information, along with glucose monitoring, to choose a variety of foods—including the ones you enjoy most.

how foods affect blood glucose

Your body needs adequate amounts of six essential nutrients to function normally. Three of these—water, vitamins, and minerals—provide no energy and do not affect blood glucose levels. The other three, carbohydrate, protein, and fat, provide your body the energy it needs to work. This energy is measured in calories. *Any* food that contains calories will cause your blood glucose levels to rise. For your body to properly use these energy calories, it needs insulin.

Whenever you eat, your food is digested and broken down into your body's primary fuel source, glucose. While all energy nutrients are broken down into glucose, carbohydrates have a more direct effect on blood glucose levels. Protein and fat have a slower, more indirect effect on those levels. Understanding this can help you predict how food will affect your glucose levels.

carbohydrates

Commonly known as sugars and starches, carbohydrates are your body's main, and preferred, source of energy. They enter your bloodstream rapidly, are fairly predictable in the way they affect glucose, and are generally completely broken down in about two hours. There are three types: simple carbohydrates, or sugars (such as table sugar and honey); digestible complex carbohydrates, or starches (in bread, pasta, and potatoes); and nondigestible complex carbohydrates, or fiber. Nearly 100 percent of the sugars and starches you eat break down into glucose; they do so at about the same speed, regardless of their source.

There are two types of simple carbohydrates, *monosaccharides* and *disaccharides*. Monosaccharides, such as glucose and fructose, are single sugar units. Disaccharides consist of two sugar units; for example, sucrose, or table sugar, is made of a glucose sugar hooked to a fructose sugar.

Digestible complex carbohydrates, or starches, are *polysaccharides*; they consist of many long chains of glucose

Types of Carbohydrates

NAME	TYPE	WHAT IT LOOKS LIKE	WHERE IT IS FOUND
glucose (dextrose)	simple monosaccharide	single glucose unit	fruits, some vegetables, honey, and corn syrup
fructose	simple monosaccharide	single fructose unit	table sugar, fruit, molasses, and honey
galactose	simple monosaccharide	single galactose unit	milk and dairy products
maltose (malt sugar)	simple disaccharide	two glucose units	produced during the breakdown of starch
sucrose (table sugar)	simple disaccharide	one glucose and one fructose unit hooked together	table sugar, fruit, vegetables, and grains
lactose (milk sugar)	simple disaccharide	one glucose and one galactose unit hooked together	milk and dairy products
starch	complex polysaccharide	long chains of glucose units hooked together	grains, legumes, and potatoes
fiber	complex polysaccharide	long chains of glucose units hooked together that the body's enzymes can't break down	fruits, vegetables, and legumes

units hooked together. Starches are found in grains, legumes, and potatoes. When starches are digested by your body, they are broken down into glucose, the simplest form of energy used by your body and your brain. The starch in a potato and the sugar in your sugar bowl, therefore, are really the same as far as your body is concerned. The body breaks down and utilizes the glucose from each in identical ways, and it has no way of knowing whether the energy originally came from a simple carbohydrate or a complex one.

However, people with diabetes often think, or have been taught, they cannot or should not have any simple carbohydrates, or sugar, in their diet. Sugar has traditionally been viewed as a forbidden or dangerous food for people with diabetes. After all, the blood "sugar" is high, so why complicate matters? Doctors and dietitians always assumed that since sugar was a simple carbohydrate, it must be more quickly digested and absorbed into the blood than more complex starches such as those in potatoes and breads. They further assumed that simple sugars would most likely cause a larger rise in blood glucose levels.

Well, doctors, dietitians, and all the food police were wrong! Multiple studies have shown that all foods increase blood sugar and that simple carbohydrates don't increase your glucose levels any higher or faster than starches alone do. In 1994, these conclusive studies led the American Diabetes Association to change its nutritional recommendations. The recommendations now say, "scientific evidence has shown that the use of sucrose as part of the meal plan does not impair blood glucose control in individuals with Type 1 or Type 2 diabetes." It is now generally recognized that the total amount of carbohydrate in your diet, not the source of the carbohydrate, is what significantly influences your blood glucose levels.

Fiber is made up mostly of complex carbohydrates—so complex, in fact, that they cannot be broken down by enzymes in your body. There are two types of fiber, soluble and insoluble. Soluble fiber remains suspended in water, while insoluble fiber does not. Soluble fiber, found in oats, barley, cereals, apples, and citrus fruits, delays glucose absorption, lowers cholesterol, and decreases the speed at which food moves through your intestines. Insoluble fiber, found in all fruits, vegetables, legumes, and seeds, also delays glucose absorption and slows the breakdown of starch, but it increases the speed at which food moves through your intestines.

protein

The second major nutrient needed by your body is protein. The protein in the foods you eat (meats, poultry, fish, beans, dairy products, and eggs) is broken down into amino acids by your body; only about 50 percent of it is eventually changed into glucose. This is a long process, however: It takes about three to five hours after a meal for the protein you have eaten to have any impact on your blood glucose. When carbohydrates and fats are not available or are in short supply (as when you don't eat between your evening meal and breakfast the next morning), amino acids can be made into glucose as a back-up source of energy for the brain and other vital organs.

fat

The third nutrient needed by your body is fat. Fat is used to maintain healthy skin and hair, to carry fat-soluble vitamins through your body, and as a major source of energy when you take in fewer calories than your body needs. Fats are changed by your body into fatty acids, which are an important source of energy for your muscles and heart. It generally takes about six to eight hours for the fat in food to be digested, and its components are released very slowly into your blood. In the end, only about 5 to 10 percent of the fat you eat is changed into glucose, so it has little direct impact on your blood glucose levels. Indirectly, however, fat does play a role in elevating blood glucose. Fat blocks the action of insulin (fatty acids increase your insulin resistance) and increases the time it takes for food to travel through your intestines. So, for example, if you eat a dinner of fried chicken, mashed potatoes, gravy, and biscuits, it may not greatly affect your glucose reading before bed. During the night, however, when this fatty, slow-moving meal finally hits your system and the fat doesn't let your insulin work very well, your blood glucose level rises. In the morning, you awaken to a whopper of a blood glucose number.

is alcohol a body fuel?

Alcohol is not a carbohydrate, protein, or fat. The body views it more as a toxin than an energy source. To your body, alcohol is a poison that needs to be broken down, detoxified, and removed from your blood as quickly as possible to prevent it from accumulating and destroying cells and organs.

When you drink, alcohol passes very quickly from your stomach and intestines into your blood without being broken down. Enzymes in your liver then do the job of breaking down the alcohol, but this process takes time. Your liver can only metabolize alcohol at a set rate, regardless of how much you have had to drink. If you drink alcohol faster than it can be broken down, it moves through your bloodstream to other parts of your body until it can be metabolized. Your brain cells are affected by this excess, impairing brain function and causing intoxication.

Whether or not you have eaten and what you have eaten are two factors that influence how quickly alcohol is absorbed into your blood. Since alcohol can only be processed at a certain rate by your liver, slowing down the absorption time (how quickly alcohol appears in your blood) can be beneficial. How fast your stomach empties into your intestines is the main control for how quickly alcohol is absorbed. The higher the fat content of a meal, the slower the emptying and the longer the absorption process. A study found that people who drank alcohol after a meal that included fat, protein, and carbohydrate absorbed the alcohol about three times more slowly than when they drank the same amount on an empty stomach.

Aside from the intoxication alcohol can cause, the process of breaking down alcohol cuts ahead of other processes on the liver's agenda. Normally, if your blood glucose level starts to drop, your liver responds by changing stored energy into glucose. This glucose then helps you avoid or slow a low blood glucose reaction. However, since your body sees alcohol as a poison, it wants to clear it from your blood as quickly as possible. In fact, it is so busy processing the alcohol, it will not make or release any glucose until the alcohol is gone from your system.

The inability to produce glucose can put you at risk for a number of different problems, including a severe hypoglycemic (low blood glucose) reaction (see the chapter Fighting Hypoglycemia). In addition, if you have consumed enough alcohol, your judgment may be impaired, decreasing or even erasing your ability to notice or recognize symptoms of hypoglycemia. To top it off, because the symptoms of hypoglycemia mimic intoxication, a low blood glucose reaction can easily be confused with drunkenness, possibly delaying emergency treatment even further should you become incoherent.

So, do you have to abstain from alcohol in order to control blood glucose? Can you have a beer with your pizza or a glass of wine with your spaghetti? There is no one right answer. You must discuss it with your diabetes care team. Your history of alcohol consumption needs to be reviewed, the medications you take need to be assessed for potential interactions with alcohol, and your diabetes control needs to be evaluated. Should you receive the okay, remember:

1. Drink only if your diabetes is under good control. Alcohol can make some diabetes problems worse. Alcohol can accumulate in nerve cells, intensifying damage from high glucose levels and worsening neuropathy. It also raises triglycerides, blood pressure, and risk of cataracts. If you have frequent hypoglycemia or a past history of severe hypoglycemia, alcohol may be too big a risk for you.

2. Drink in moderation. The breakdown of alcohol by your liver is a slow process, so the amount of alcohol you drink needs to be controlled to prevent intoxication. Moderation generally means no more than two drinks per day for men and no more than one per day for women. A single drink is defined as 12 ounces of beer, 5 ounces of wine, or

1 ½ ounces of distilled liquor. Remember, alcohol has no nutrients, only calories, most of which your body stores as fat.

3. Do not skip a meal or decrease your food intake when drinking. Have your drink with a meal or shortly after eating. Never drink on an empty stomach, and do not skip meals or substitute alcohol for your usual meal or snack.

4. Always carry a form of identification, preferably one that indicates you have diabetes. This lets people know that your erratic behavior or loss of consciousness may not be due to intoxication but rather to severe hypoglycemia.

5. Never drink alone. Inform those around you that you have diabetes, and teach them the signs and symptoms of hypoglycemia. This way, they will not confuse these symptoms of hypoglycemia with intoxication and ignore or delay treatment of a possible hypoglycemic reaction.

6. Remain sober. Since alcohol has a relaxing effect, it can impair your judgment. You need to eat your meals, take your medication, and test your blood sugar on schedule.

7. Test your blood glucose frequently. Understand how alcohol affects you by testing prior to drinking, after drinking, and the next day. Be sure to always test your blood glucose before going to sleep. And never give yourself extra insulin or take extra diabetes pills to treat a high blood glucose reading just before going to bed. You could become dangerously hypoglycemic as you sleep and never even notice it.

what about sweeteners?

There are two types of sweeteners on the market today, those that have calories, called nutritive sweeteners, and those that have no calories, called artificial, or nonnutritive, sweeteners. Only the nutritive sweeteners affect blood glucose directly, but you'll still need to note the other ingredients in foods that use artificial sweeteners.

nutritive sweeteners. The simple carbohydrates sucrose and fructose are the most common nutritive sweeteners used; both contribute calories and influence your blood glucose levels.

Sugar alcohols, also called polyols, contain calories and carbohydrates and are often used as substitute sweeteners, especially in candy. While the name implies two seemingly forbidden words, sugar and alcohol, sugar alcohols are neither sugars nor alcoholic substances in the common sense of the term. (The scientific definition of alcohol is simply "a processed liquid.") Sugar alcohols are the commercially produced, processed liquids from sucrose, glucose, and starches (polysaccharides).

They also occur naturally in plants such as fruits and berries. Common sugar alcohols include sorbitol, mannitol, maltitol, and xylitol.

Another sugar alcohol, called *hydrogenated starch hydrolysate,* is made by partially breaking down corn, wheat, or potato starch and then adding hydrogens, at a high temperature and under pressure, to the partially broken-down mixture. As a result, it contains higher quantities of hydrogenated polysaccharides as well as sorbitol, mannitol, maltitol, and xylitol. It is kind of the "complex carbohydrate" of the sugar alcohols, used in a variety of products, especially sugar-free candies, because it does not crystallize. It also blends well with flavors and can be used with low-calorie sweeteners.

As a group, sugar alcohols are not completely absorbed and used by your body, so they contribute fewer calories and carbohydrates than the same amount of other nutritive sweeteners, such as sucrose. For this reason, they are referred to as reduced-energy or low-energy sweeteners. But because they are not completely absorbed, they can produce unpleasant side effects, such as diarrhea, bloating, and gas, when consumed in excess.

artificial sweeteners. Artificial sweeteners are man-made, intensely sweet products most commonly used in reduced-calorie foods and beverages. They are termed nonnutritive sweeteners because they add very few, if any, calories and carbohydrates to foods. Because such a small amount of these sweeteners is needed to produce a "sweet" taste in foods, they are also referred to as high-intensity sweeteners. The major artificial sweeteners are NutraSweet (aspartame), Sweet One (acesulfame K), Splenda (sucralose), and Sweet'N Low (saccharin).

"sugar-free" products. How is it that a manufacturer can slap a big "Sugar Free" label on the front of a box of cookies even though the product contains sugar? The answers: "Quite simply" and "quite legally." All that the term "sugar free" means is that a product contains less than .5 gram of sugar in a serving—and "sugar" in this context is defined as sucrose. That's right. "Sugar free" simply means that table sugar or cane sugar is not in the item. The manufacturer can add fructose and any other nutritive sweetener and still call it "sugar free."

As a result, it is not unusual for a sugar-free product to actually contain more total carbohydrates than the regular version of the same product. For the person with diabetes, that means the sugar-free item will actually raise blood glucose *more* than the regular version of the food would. The same applies for many fat-free foods. They truly have less than .5 gram of fat per serving, but when the fat is removed, simple carbohydrates may be added instead. So some fat-free

SWEETENERS

nutritive (calorie-containing) sweeteners

sucrose (white sugar)	It is very versatile in terms of use, readily available, and inexpensive.
glucose	It has limited use because of a lower level of sweetness and is mainly used in candies to provide smoothness at high temperatures.
fructose	It is sweeter than sucrose in cold liquids, but in warm liquids and solid foods, it is only as sweet as sucrose. It enhances fruit flavors.
honey	It is nutritionally similar to sucrose and is chemically formed from nectar by bees. It has a very distinctive flavor and a very high water content.
lactose	It is the sugar found in milk and is a disaccharide, made up of glucose and galactose linked together. It has a very low sweetness, which limits its uses, but it is often used in combination with intense sweeteners as a "filler." Lactose intolerance is common and occurs in people who lack the digestive enzyme lactase, which breaks apart the glucose and galactose units.
sorbitol, mannitol	They are sugar alcohols and are about half as sweet as sucrose, which limits their uses. They are incompletely absorbed by your body, so they add fewer calories and carbohydrates to the food being eaten. Because of incomplete digestion, they can cause diarrhea, gas, and bloating when used in large quantities. They are more expensive than sucrose.
xylitol, maltitol	They are sugar alcohols. Both are about as sweet as sucrose and so are more widely used, especially in candies and baked goods. They are incompletely absorbed, so they have fewer calories and carbohydrates. Large quantities may cause diarrhea, gas, and bloating.
hydrogenated starch hydrolysate	It's the "complex carbohydrate" of sugar alcohols. It's made of large chains of polysaccharides plus hydrogen put together under heat and pressure to form very stable, complex sugar alcohols. Widely used in candies and with low-calorie, nonnutritive sweeteners.

nonnutritive (calorie-free) sweeteners

saccharin (Sweet'N Low)	It provides no energy. It is 200 to 700 times sweeter than sucrose but has a bitter, metallic aftertaste.
aspartame (NutraSweet)	It is made up of two amino acids linked together. The amino acids break apart when they are heated, and the sweetness deteriorates, so it can only be used in cold foods and drinks. It is 160 to 220 times sweeter than sucrose. It cannot be used by persons with phenylketonuria.
acesulfame K (Sweet One)	It is an organic salt consisting of carbon, nitrogen, oxygen, hydrogen, sulphur, and potassium atoms. It is 200 times sweeter than sucrose and is heat stable.
sucralose (Splenda)	It is the only nonnutritive sweetener made from sugar. Through a special method, three hydrogen-oxygen groups on the sugar molecule are replaced with three chlorines. It is used as a sugar replacement and an additive in various desserts, confections, and nonalcoholic beverages. It is 600 times sweeter than sucrose. Its sweetening power is not reduced with heating.

and some fat-free/sugar-free products actually have more carbohydrates and will raise blood glucose levels higher than the regular item would.

Also understand that a sugar-free food is not always calorie free, low in calories, or low in simple carbohydrates. Some foods may even have sugar listed on the label, even though they fit the legal definition of "sugar free." Milk is a good example. On the food label for milk, you will find that one serving contains 13 grams of sugar. Milk doesn't contain sucrose, or table sugar. It does, however, contain the naturally occurring simple carbohydrate (sugar) called lactose. The point is that because a product is labeled "sugar free" doesn't mean you can ignore its potential effect on your blood glucose levels.

check that label!

It's important to look closely at the nutrition label on a food to find the actual calorie and carbohydrate counts. As you look at any product, the middle part of the nutrition label contains information on carbohydrate, fat, protein, and other nutrients. This section has the greatest amount of information for the person with diabetes who is trying to analyze the connection between food and glucose levels.

On all labels, carbohydrates are measured in grams. As you've learned, gram for gram, all carbohydrates have the same effect on blood sugar levels. So use the food labels to compare foods in terms of their total carbohydrate as well as their fiber content. Make sure the serving sizes you are comparing are similar. Then choose the product that best fits into your carbohydrate goals (which you'll learn about shortly). In addition, monitoring your blood sugar before and after eating or drinking will help you to see a food's effect on your blood sugar.

carbs are key

Okay, so now you have a basic understanding of how the nutrients in food affect your blood glucose. To successfully use this knowledge as part of your diabetes self-care, you need to make personal food choices that are compatible with your blood glucose goals and your tastes. Since carbohydrates obviously have the greatest direct effect on glucose levels, determining the amount of carbohydrates that your body can manage well is a cornerstone in your glucose management. It's simple, really. But before you begin, you should take a close look at your perceptions, preconceptions, and habits regarding food and eating; they can make eating much more complicated than need be. Adjusting them can allow you to enjoy the freedom that simplicity brings—and allow you to enjoy eating while you control your diabetes.

don't stereotype your carbs

According to multiple studies, the *amount* of digestible carbohydrate in what you eat is more important than the *type* (sugar or starch) in terms of blood glucose. In other words, a carbohydrate is a carbohydrate. While a snack of one large, extra-chunky chocolate chip cookie may seem "bad" and a snack of three small sugar-free cookies may seem "good," your body can't tell the difference between them if both snacks have the same amount of digestible carbohydrate. Both will raise your glucose level the same amount.

You may be thinking, "No way." You may have preconceptions telling you that eating an extra-chunky cookie or a candy bar must raise your glucose levels higher than eating, say, a baked potato or even a few sugar-free cookies. Perhaps your experience seems to back you up. The culprit in this apparent discrepancy, though, is not the type of carbohydrate. Your preconceptions—and the total amount of carbohydrate you consume—are much more likely to blame.

Consider this: Generally, when, what, and why you eat has as much (or more) to do with habit or craving as it has to do with hunger. So while you may eat just one baked potato, you may be driven to eat an entire candy bar, not because you are still hungry after finishing half of it, but because it just tastes so good and perhaps it has

SOME OF THE FOODS THAT CONTAIN CARBOHYDRATE:		
rice	pasta	breads
cereals	fruits	juices
vegetables	milk & milk products	nuts
candy	cakes	pies
chips & pretzels	beans	popcorn
crackers	soda	pancakes & waffles
tortillas	cookies	jams & jellies
FOODS THAT DO NOT HAVE CARBOHYDRATE:		
meats and fats		

been a long time since you've allowed yourself to have chocolate. You may even feel that, because it's been so long, you are entitled to two candy bars. So you end up eating more candy—and more total carbohydrate. It's that larger amount of carbohydrate, not the source of the carbohydrate, that sends your glucose soaring.

The kind of deprivation that might drive you to eat a second candy bar can drive your eating in other ways as well. There's nothing that can heighten your desire for a food quite like being told you cannot have it. So, you have a nice lunch, followed by a sugar-free cookie—followed by three extra-chunky chocolate chip cookies. You figure you've eaten what you were supposed to eat, it's only fair that you get to eat what you really want in return. You then blame your elevated glucose levels on the extra-chunky cookies. While they are a contributor, they are not the problem. If you had ended your lunch with one of the extra-chunky cookies you wanted in the first place, rather than the sugar-free one you were "supposed to have," your glucose level would have been lower in the end. It was your drive to get what you want, and your initial self-imposed deprivation, that set you up to fail big time. It's this kind of restrictive thinking that can make some foods seem off-limits or more dangerous in terms of glucose control. And it's this kind of restrictive thinking that can make you feel deprived, triggering, in turn, unhealthful eating behaviors that end up defeating your best intentions.

Deprivation can also lead to desperation, and desperate times lead to desperate measures. For example, perhaps you're always the last one in your household to go to bed, staying up well past the others because you're "just not tired yet." Or perhaps you decline dinner invitations and evenings out because you are "too tired"; you send everyone else out, leaving you home, alone. Now, in quiet solitude, you can eat in peace, without anyone commenting or watching your intake. You're like the escaped convict, trying to outrun the law before you are captured again by the food police and thrown back into deprivation jail.

These types of preconceptions and dysfunctional eating habits can also interfere with your dietary diabetes management. Food habits and eating patterns are developed over years and are often ingrained from childhood. You do something one way because that is just how it is done. You clean your plate because you shouldn't waste food. You eat every last bit of food because you paid for it or it is free. You eat because the label on your pill bottle says you must take it with food. You eat because the clock tells you it's time. These food-related habits have very little to do with hunger or your glucose levels, but they have become the rules that drive your eating.

To end this cycle of deprivation and dysfunctional eating and be able to truly use your food choices to help control your diabetes, you need to make all food equal and make no food off-limits. You need to convince yourself once and for all that there are no such things as good foods and bad foods. There are merely foods that affect your blood glucose in different ways. This will eliminate your feelings of deprivation. If you know you can have candy whenever you want, the drive to eat it like it was going out of style will disappear. You'll be able to eat because you are hungry for a certain item, not because you'll never have it again.

Instead of eating because you want to or are supposed to, ask yourself instead if you are hungry. You have an internal wisdom that lets you know when you need to eat and when you need to stop. While this system has many triggers, one is your blood glucose level. When your blood glucose is on the low side, you become hungry; when it's higher, hunger is absent. (If you find yourself having to eat when you're not hungry because you need to take your medication with food, discuss this fact with your diabetes care team.) Eliminating the deprivation and examining your habits will let you find the carbohydrate balance that allows you to maintain your glucose goals. It will help you change your relationship with food for the better and improve your diabetes control. It may even enhance your ability to battle other aspects of Syndrome X, such as overweight and high blood cholesterol.

explore and experiment

To gain a more detailed and concrete understanding of how you can use your food choices to control your blood sugar levels, you must pay attention to how individual foods act in your body. You need to approach this just as a scientist would, collecting data about blood glucose and types and amounts of foods, then drawing conclusions that are based on that data.

The first step is for you to eat absolutely normally. Eat what you want, when you want it, in whatever amount you desire. Use the Nutrient Counter in this book or check food labels to determine which of those foods contain carbohydrate, then keep a running tally of the total grams of carbohydrate you eat throughout the entire day. Take detailed, honest notes.

Along with taking these notes, you need to test your blood glucose levels. Testing will allow you to see how well your insulin level (either that you have injected or that your body has pro-

IT'S NOT WHAT YOU'RE EATING, IT'S HOW MUCH YOU'RE EATING

45 grams of carbohydrates	amount you would normally eat	amount of carbohydrates actually eaten
2 baked potatoes	1 potato—reasonable, standard, accepted amount	23
1 regular-sized candy bar	2 candy bars—one because you crave it and one because you've blown your diet anyway, so you might as well go for it	90
3 pieces of whole-wheat toast	2 pieces of toast—because the toaster holds two slices. In addition, you have to finish the second piece because "there are children starving somewhere."	30
1½ cups of a sugar-frosted cereal	3 cups—Who decided that ¾ of a cup of cereal was a serving size? In a country where we "super size" everything, small is sure to leave me hungry.	90

duced) matches your carbohydrate intake. No matter its source, insulin works with the food you eat. It is this balance that is a key aspect of diabetes control. If you eat too much food for the insulin that is available, your glucose level will be too high; if you eat too little, your glucose level will be too low.

Test before you eat and then one, two, three, and four hours after the meal. As a general guideline, aim for a pre-meal glucose goal of 90–130 mg/dl; one hour after the meal, less than 180 mg/dl; two hours after the meal, less than 160 mg/dl; three hours after, less than 140; and at four hours, or prior to your next meal, back to 90–130 mg/dl. Just as you know the number of miles per gallon (mpg) of gas you can travel in your car, you will gradually begin to figure out your body's *cpm,* or *carbohydrates per*

meal—the "distance" your body can go each time you eat a certain amount of carbohydrates.

You may find that eating foods that contain only carbohydrates causes your blood glucose to rise rapidly or stay too high after the meal. Carbohydrates in combination with varying amounts of fat and/or protein will affect your blood glucose differently. In addition, you may discover that high-fat foods elevate your blood glucose levels as well.

It is important to know that any food has the ability to make blood sugar levels rise, but different types of food as well as different amounts will result in different levels of blood sugar in your body. You may find that over-eating (eating when you are not hungry) makes blood sugar levels increase rapidly and stay too high. Overeating may not allow insulin to do its job properly. If you listen to your body's internal hunger cues and respect the

Note: It is fine to use total carbohydrate values to figure your CPM. Subtracting out the amount of fiber, which does not raise blood glucose, from each food item can be complicated and time consuming; in addition, for many food items, the fiber content is not available or listed on the packaging. Whichever method you choose, it is probably best to be consistent, using either total carbs or total carbs minus fiber for your calculations.

FIGURE YOUR CPM (CARBS* PER MEAL) RATE

What you ate (Specify the foods you ate and the amount of carbohydrates.)	blood glucose start 90–130	1 hour <180	2 hours <160	3 hours <140	4 hours 90–130

feeling of fullness, you'll find that your blood glucose will rise more slowly and peak at a lower level. Insulin, in turn, will be able to do its job properly and keep blood sugars at a healthy level. This type of balanced eating helps control diabetes and helps you feel better.

As you experiment and test your blood glucose, try a wide variety of foods. Enjoy different types of carbohydrates, from pasta to potatoes, biscuits to green beans, and bread to blueberries. Eat a variety of proteins, from eggs to cheese and ground turkey to prime rib. Try various types of fats, from butter to margarine and sour cream to mayonnaise. Look for patterns in the ways various foods and food combinations affect your glucose.

Eating a wide variety of foods will also help ensure that you get the nutrients you need—not just the carbohydrate, protein, and fat but also the vitamins and minerals that are essential to overall good health. In addition, the multitudes of tastes, textures, and colors will continue to enhance your eating pleasure and help prevent the feelings of deprivation that can lead to bingeing and overeating.

listen to your body

There truly is an alternative to diets, those externally imposed, dictatorial dietary restrictions that result in those overpowering cravings and abandon-ment of self-care. Work to understand the effect of foods on your blood glucose levels. Know that restricting foods creates "good" and "bad" food and that these terms imply guilt and assign emotional labels to food.

Learn how you use food for comfort and calming. When you catch yourself eating when you're not hungry, ask yourself why. What do you really need? Do you need a break from that project? Would a walk, a bath, a call to a friend, or some quiet time make you feel better? Are you craving the food because you've been trying to stay away from it? Listen to your thoughts. Then listen to your body; it knows what it needs.

Part III of this book, which includes the Nutrient Counter, will help you expand your food horizons. With more foods to choose from, you'll find it much easier to select foods that match your carbohydrate needs and please your taste buds. Part III also includes advice on choosing foods that not only fit into your diabetes care plan but can improve your health and help you temper other risk factors such as excess weight, high blood pressure, and high blood cholesterol. So let food be both your joy and your remedy.

moving toward better control

The three cornerstones in the treatment of diabetes are food, medications, and activity. Of these three, activity is often a first choice for the person who has diabetes. Moving toward a more physically active life is generally inexpensive, convenient, and easy and usually produces great rewards in terms of blood glucose control and a general feeling of well-being.

If you recall, whenever you actively use a muscle, you burn both fatty acids and glucose. During and after periods of activity, your falling glucose level is sensed by the beta cells in your pancreas, and they relax their output of insulin. This gives your beta cells a break from excessive insulin production. In addition, the lower insulin levels signal your liver to empty its glucose reserves (glycogen) into the blood to supply the muscles with needed energy. As physical activity continues, the liver converts amino acids, lactic acid, and fats into glucose to supply the muscles. If the activity

continues long enough, even the body's fat cells get in the game. They compensate for the reduced fatty acid levels in your blood by converting their stored triglycerides into fatty acids.

When all of these steps are considered, it's easy to see why using your muscles is the perfect treatment for diabetes. It lowers blood glucose, lowers fatty acid levels in your blood, and reduces the workload of your pancreas. And, unless you are on a medication that can cause hypoglycemia, physical activity won't cause your blood glucose level to fall below normal the way some other diabetes treatments may.

before you get going

Becoming more physically active is not completely without risks for people with diabetes. (On the other hand, remaining sedentary is no bargain, either; it does nothing to help your glucose control, your weight management, or your overall well-being.) To gain the benefits of increased physical activity and minimize potential risks, you need to understand and evaluate those risks up front and take steps to prevent problems before they occur.

hypoglycemia

For people with diabetes who take medication or insulin, hypoglycemia is a concern. Whenever you are physically active, your muscles burn glucose. First, they gobble up the glucose they have stored as glycogen. As the activity continues, glucose from the blood pours into the muscles to supply their energy needs, lowering blood glucose levels. This march of glucose from the blood into the muscles doesn't end when the activity stops, however. The body needs to refill the muscles' glucose storage tanks in preparation for future movement. As a result, a hypoglycemic reaction can occur not only during periods of activity but up to 24 hours later.

Some people with diabetes who have frequently experienced hypoglycemia begin to associate any form of activity with a loss of glucose control. For such individuals, a lack of glucose testing may keep them in the dark about how their body reacts to activity. As a result, they are unprepared for the low blood glucose level that can occur when they mow the lawn or when they take a brisk walk through the park. When such a low occurs, they may grab a handful of jelly beans to treat the low, only to find their glucose level skyrocketing as a result. So they take extra insulin or medication at dinner to treat the high, but the blood-glucose roller-coaster ride continues with another low before they go to bed. These fluctuations create great confusion and frustration, leaving these individuals upset and scared. Activity, they may decide, is not worth the seemingly unpredictable swings in glucose. For such individuals, more frequent blood glucose testing can help them better understand their body's response to exercise and prepare for it by adjusting medication or food intake. (You'll find advice on such adjustments later in this chapter.)

heart disease

Before you increase your activity level, you need to consider the possible presence of heart disease. As you've already learned, coronary heart disease is very common in people with diabetes, affecting perhaps as many as 50 percent of them. To assess your risk, you and your doctor need to take into account your age, your blood pressure, your blood fats, whether you have protein in your urine, the length of time you have had diabetes, and your family history. So before you begin increasing your level of activity, consult your doctor and, if appropriate, have an exercise tolerance test. This test is done on a treadmill and reflects your heart's ability to work under stress. Your chances of having a positive result, indicating heart disease, increase with each risk factor you have. Even if you are at increased risk

Benefits of being more active
- Lower blood glucose
- Lower blood pressure
- Lower blood fats
- Better cardiovascular (heart and lung) fitness
- Weight loss and/or maintenance
- Improved sense of well-being

Assess your risk before you start

Before starting moderate- to high-intensity activity, you should have an exercise stress test if you:
- are older than 35
- are older than 25 and have had type 2 diabetes for more than 10 years or type 1 for more than 15 years
- have protein in your urine
- have high blood pressure
- have high blood cholesterol
- have a family history of heart disease

Talk to your doctor about having a stress test if *any* of the above applies to you.

or have a positive test, you will likely still be able to increase your physical activity; you will just need to work more closely with your diabetes care team to set safe guidelines for activity and, perhaps, to determine if medications to lower your risk of heart trouble are in order.

diabetes complications

Before you increase your activity level, you need to account for any diabetic complications or related conditions that may be present. Some types of activity may not be wise for people with certain medical conditions.

Any activity that includes straining, such as weight lifting, can dramatically increase blood pressure during the actual activity, further aggravating any hypertension that is present. To lessen any potential problems, you need to have your blood pressure well controlled before you start increasing your activity level and especially before beginning an activity that involves straining.

Proliferative retinopathy is also aggravated by straining, which increases the pressure within some of the weakened blood vessels of the eyes. Activities that require straining or that involve jarring or rapid head motions may also cause an acute hemorrhage in already weakened eye vessels. For this reason, it is important to have your eyes examined for signs

of retinopathy before starting an exercise program and have them rechecked annually.

If you have significant nerve disease in your feet, you may not be able to feel injuries to your feet, the most common of which are blisters. This does not mean you cannot exercise, but it means that you need to have your feet checked by your doctor first and you must observe good foot care at home, including inspecting your feet for sore spots and minor injuries daily. You'll also want to get expert advice on proper footwear for the activity and be sure that the footwear you choose is fitted properly to your feet.

guidelines for activity

The following guidelines can help you increase your activity level safely. Be sure to work with your diabetes care team, too, so they can monitor you and provide specialized advice for your specific situation.

screening

First, be screened by your doctor for any possible problems before you start any type of activity. This exam should include a treadmill test for people with diabetes who fit certain criteria (see "Assess Your Risk Before You Start"), an eye examination for proliferative retinopathy, a urine examination for protein, and a medical evaluation of your feet.

type of activity

Once you've received your team's okay for exercise, you need to choose activities that fit your physical condition, lifestyle, and tastes. Many people with diabetes, especially those who have not been physically active for a while, find that easy, low-impact activities such as walking and swimming are perfect.

Whatever you choose, make sure the activities are enjoyable for you and take into account your abilities and condition. The activities don't even have to be "exercises" in the traditional sense, as long as they get you moving. Square dancing, taking your dog on long walks, riding your bike, gardening, and even walking the golf course all count. Vary them so you don't get bored and fall prey to easy excuses. Choose some that can be done with others and some that can be done alone; some that can be done indoors, some that can be done outdoors; some that can be done when your schedule is light, and some that can be fit in when you're strapped for time.

time, intensity, and duration

Begin each exercise session with a five- to ten-minute period of low-intensity warm-up activity (such as marching in place) and gentle stretching. The warm-up will prepare your heart for increased activity. The stretching will help you avoid tendon and muscle

problems, which are common in people whose tendons have become brittle after years of high blood glucose levels.

After you warm up and stretch, start the aerobic portion of your activity. An aerobic activity is one that works the large muscles—those in the legs and buttocks or arms and shoulders—continuously for an extended period of time. In so doing, it increases your body's demand for oxygen, forcing both your breathing and heart rate to speed up.

One way to determine how hard your body should work during physical activity is to use something called a target heart rate range.

WHAT'S YOUR TARGET RANGE?

INTENSITY	% MAX HEART RATE*
very light	<35
light	35–54
moderate	55–70
hard	71–90
very hard	>90
maximal	100

*maximal heart rate = 220 – age

FIGURING YOUR TARGET RANGE

For a moderately intense (55–70% max) activity level:
[220 – (your age)]×.55 to [220 – (your age)]×.70

EXAMPLE

Target heart rate range for 54-year-old doing moderately intense activity:
[220 – 54]×.55 to [220 – 54]×.70
91 to 116 beats per minute

To help establish your target range, you need to first determine your maximal heart rate. To calculate this number, simply subtract your age from 220. The high and low ends of your appropriate target heart rate range will be percentages of this number. For example, you might aim for the moderate intensity range, which is between 55 and 70 percent of your maximal heart rate. *It is important, however, to work with your diabetes care team to determine the intensity range that is most appropriate for you.* You will also want to ask for specific advice regarding how often and how long you should exercise. During the exercise, to determine if you are working in your target range, you will need to occasionally check your heart rate. To do this, count the number of heartbeats (by feeling the pulse on the inner side of your wrist) for six seconds and add a zero to the end of that number; that's the number of times your heart is beating per minute. And that's the number that should stay in your target range during the aerobic activity.

It's always best to increase physical activity slowly and build up gradually. If you find it uncomfortable to exercise near the higher end of your target range, talk to your diabetes care team. They will probably suggest that you shoot for a lower intensity but a longer duration. As time passes, you'll be able to maintain a higher and higher level of activity for longer and longer periods of time.

Regardless of the activity you choose, you should end each workout period with ten minutes of cool-down and more gentle stretching. You want to slowly decrease the pace of your activity for several minutes rather than stop abruptly. You also want to take advantage of the fact that your muscles are warmed up to do some gentle stretching.

If you try to do some extra activity every other day, you will be amazed at the difference in your glucose control. Get moving every day, and the benefits will be even greater.

avoiding glucose problems

To preempt problems with your glucose levels during exercise, there are a number of things you can do:

- Plan your activity to follow a meal so that it can help lower the increased blood glucose level that follows eating.
- Check your blood glucose 30 minutes before and then just prior to activity. This way you can see which direction your glucose level is heading and anticipate a low in time to take preventive action.
- If you are at risk for hypoglycemia, plan for a possible hypoglycemic

episode. Carry glucose tablets with you; if symptoms of low blood glucose develop (see the chapter Fighting Hypoglycemia to learn how to recognize a low), stop the activity immediately and use the fast-acting glucose.

- If you manage your diabetes with insulin, know the peak time of your insulin and plan your activities accordingly. Avoiding the times when your insulin is peaking and at its strongest will help you prevent hypoglycemia.

- When injecting insulin, avoid the muscle areas that you will be using during the activity. For example, if you will be playing tennis, avoid using your racket arm and even, perhaps, your legs for your injection at the meal prior to your game. Most people find the abdomen or the buttocks work best before exercise.

- When planning to be extremely active, test your glucose level prior to getting started. If your blood glucose is near normal but you have the potential to develop hypoglycemia, you will need to eat prior to the activity. (If you take insulin, you will either need to eat prior to the activity or lower your insulin dose.)

- If your blood glucose before the activity is more than 250 mg/dl, check your urine for ketones. If they are present, activity will actually cause your blood glucose level to

increase. An elevated glucose level and positive ketones indicate that your diabetes is uncontrolled and you need to contact your diabetes care team for advice immediately.

- Monitor your glucose during exercise to see what effect activity has on you. Check it every half hour during exercise and again when you are finished.

- Be sure to drink plenty of fluids. Sweating means you are losing fluids that need to be replaced. Water is usually a great choice.

- If, during any activity, you ever experience shortness of breath, chest pain, or leg cramps that go away with rest, contact your doctor immediately. These are all possible signs of blocked arteries and require an evaluation by your doctor.

- If you repeatedly experience episodes of hypoglycemia during and/or after increased levels of activity, you should contact your doctor and discuss the possibility of a change in your medications.

One final thought: Being active needs to be fun. Otherwise, you're much less likely to stick with an active lifestyle. So, choose your activities accordingly, then go out and play at least a little every day.

using pills to treat diabetes

Be intolerant!

Always remember that high glucose levels are extremely toxic. Your body cannot tolerate them—nor should you. Don't count your prescriptions and feel that you've failed. It is not the number of pills you take, but rather the glucose levels you achieve, the complications you prevent, and the joyful life you lead that determine your treatment success.

For many people who have type 2 diabetes, using food and activity to control blood glucose is not enough. For them, oral diabetes medications can be lifesavers—helping to lower their blood glucose levels and stave off diabetes complications.

have I failed?

Imagine yourself sailing down a highway at 60 miles per hour. It is a flat, open road, and you require a steady amount of fuel to keep you at this speed. Then you hit a mountain range. Maintaining your speed as you begin to ascend requires more and more fuel—you must press farther down on the gas pedal to maintain a speed of 60 miles per hour. The disease of diabetes is similar in a way. When first diagnosed, you may be able to maintain a steady speed, or steady glucose range, with a few modifications in your lifestyle. However, the disease of diabetes has mountains built into its route—it is

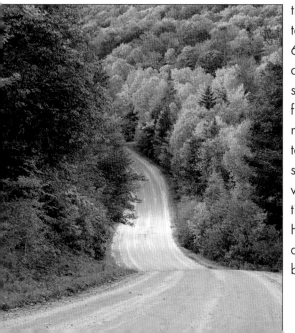

a progressive, "uphill" disease that requires more and more "fuel" to keep your speed within your target range.

In general, the first steps taken to move your glucose levels back toward normal are to increase the level of activity in your life and to change your relationship with food. Sometimes these steps can't lower your glucose levels enough to reach a normal range or, over time, they may not continue to keep your level within your target range. You may then require medication to help you achieve or maintain your target glucose levels. If and when this happens, do not look at the use of medications as a failure on your part in any way. Keep in mind that diabetes is a chronic, progressive disease that requires more and more treatments to keep blood glucose under the same good control. Your goal, in the end, should not be to avoid medications but to avoid complications. Fortunately, recent years have seen the advent of several new and effective treatments that can help you reach that goal.

how do pills work?

People with type 1 diabetes make very little, if any, insulin, so they are dependent on insulin injections to keep them alive. Since the pills used to treat diabetes are not the same as insulin and do not contain any insulin, they are of no use to people with type 1 diabetes. The pills used to treat diabetes can lower blood glucose levels, but only in people with type 2 diabetes whose bodies still make some insulin but just don't use it well enough.

To understand how pills treat diabetes, you must first understand why your blood glucose levels are still high. For you and others with type 2 diabetes, your difficulties with glucose control appear to stem from no fewer than three areas. First, your muscles are not taking up the glucose in your bloodstream. Second, the liver is over-producing glucose, further increasing the glucose levels in your blood. And third, the insulin production by your pancreas cannot keep up with the high levels of glucose.

In this gradual system breakdown, the primary problem seems to be insulin resistance in your muscles. Your muscles are not responding to your insulin, and so the glucose is not being taken in by your muscles; instead, the glucose builds up in your blood. It's as if each of your cells is in its own room, with the radio blasting. Insulin and glucose are both at the door, insulin knocking as hard as it can, but because the radio is up so loud, the cell cannot hear it.

The next problem lies in your liver. Your liver normally stops pumping out glucose when it "sees" insulin in your blood. When you eat, your glucose level rises, which prompts the release of insulin from your pancreas. The insulin's job is to get the muscle cells to take in the glucose. When your liver sees the insulin, it knows that glucose has entered the system, so it stops releasing its own glucose stores. The insulin levels in your body normally decrease when your glucose levels drop, such as when you fast overnight or when it has been longer than four hours since you have eaten. Your liver does not see as much insulin, so it kicks into gear and begins to make glucose to keep your levels in a normal range. When your liver cells become insulin resistant, however, they cannot see the insulin, and therefore they think, wrongly, that your glucose levels are low. So your liver pumps out more glucose despite the fact that there's already glucose in the bloodstream waiting to get into your muscle cells.

The last and crucial problem is the inability of your pancreas, specifically the beta cells in your pancreas, to make enough insulin to keep up with this resistance. As glucose and fatty acids build up in your bloodstream, your beta cells must pump out excessive amounts of insulin to keep up; eventually, this excessive demand seems to poison the beta cells, and they begin to die off. When you reach a point where there are very few beta cells still living, your blood glucose level increases greatly, which further hampers the body's ability to take up glucose, causing the extremely elevated blood glucose levels that are seen in uncontrolled diabetes.

The pills available to treat the elevated glucose levels of diabetes work on these three problem areas. They stimulate your beta cells to make more insulin, they decrease your liver's glucose production, and they make your muscle cells more sensitive to glucose. While most people who have type 2 diabetes still make some insulin, it is not enough to control glucose levels. The medications help the body make enough insulin available to control the glucose levels.

The oral diabetes medications available today fall into five different categories: sulfonylureas, biguanides, alpha-glucosidase inhibitors, thiazo-lidinediones (glitazones), and glitinides. The five types have different actions and support your body in different ways. As you and your diabetes care team begin to consider one or more of these pills to help keep your glucose levels in a healthy range, make sure you stay completely informed. Know the names of all of your medications, how much you need to take, and when to take them. Be aware of any possible side effects and whether or not they can be taken with any other medications you currently take. The following discussions can help you become familiar with the medications available.

sulfonylureas

The *sulfonylureas* (sul-fa-nul-ur-ee-ahs) are the original diabetes pills; they were the first pills ever available to treat diabetes. Prior to their introduction, insulin was the only treatment for elevated glucose levels. Around the time of World War II, it was noticed that antibacterial agents called sulfa drugs also seemed to lower blood glucose. But it wasn't until the 1950s that this discovery would lead to the introduction in the United States of sulfalike drugs, the sulfonylureas, for the treatment of diabetes.

Sulfonylureas work by stimulating your pancreas to release more insulin. The first medication that was available in this category is called Orinase (known generically as tolbutamide); it was followed shortly by Diabinese (chlorpropamide) and Tolinase (tolazamide). These medications are often referred to as "first generation sulfonylureas," since they were the first pills released in this category. Since the 1950s, newer and stronger sulfonylureas have been released. These include the "second generation sulfonylureas" Diabeta, Micronase, Glynase (all brand names for glyburide), Glu-

NEWER SULFONYLUREAS IN A NUTSHELL

BRAND NAME	GENERIC NAME	TYPICAL DAILY DOSE	MAXIMUM DAILY DOSE	DURATION OF ACTION
Micronase, Diabeta	glyburide	1.25–20 mg Taken as a single or divided dose, once or twice a day	20 mg	24 hours
Glynase	micronized glyburide	1.5–6 mg Taken as a single dose, once a day	6 mg	24 hours
Glucotrol	glipizide	5–20 mg Taken as a single dose, once or twice a day	20 mg	12–24 hours
Glucotrol XL	extended-release glipizide	5–20 mg Taken as a single dose, once a day	20 mg	24 hours
Amaryl	glimepiride	1–8 mg Taken as a single or divided dose, once or twice a day	8 mg	24 hours

OLDER SULFONYLUREAS IN A NUTSHELL

BRAND NAME	GENERIC NAME	TYPICAL DAILY DOSE	MAXIMUM DAILY DOSE	DURATION OF ACTION
Orinase	tolbutamide	250–3,000 mg Taken as a divided dose, twice a day	3,000 mg	6–12 hours
Tolinase	tolazamide	100–1,000 mg Taken as a single or divided dose, once or twice a day	1,000 mg	24 hours
Diabinese	chlorpropamide	100–750 mg Taken as a single dose, once a day	750 mg	24–72 hours

cotrol, and Glucotrol XL (both brand names of glipizide), as well as the more recently introduced "third generation sulfonylurea" Amaryl (glimepiride).

The sulfonylureas all operate by the same mechanism. They work on your beta cells, pushing them to make more insulin in order to lower your glucose level. Because of your insulin resistance, you require substantially more insulin than a non–insulin-resistant person to get the same amount of glucose into cells. In other words, it takes more insulin to keep your glucose levels normal just as it takes more gas in your car's tank to travel the same distance.

These pills help by lowering your blood glucose levels, but because they continually work on your pancreas, they cause insulin to be released even when it may not be needed. This is the major drawback, and major side effect, of all the sulfonylurea medications: They can cause hypoglycemia, or low blood glucose (see the chapter Fighting Hypoglycemia for more detailed information). Other side effects, although uncommon, include skin rashes, dark urine, stomach upset, and an increased sensitivity to the sun.

Diabinese, a first generation sulfonylurea, has a longer duration of action in the body than the newer medications. With this very prolonged duration comes a greater risk of extended and severe hypoglycemia under certain conditions. Diabinese can also cause additional side effects including hyponatremia (low sodium in the blood) and a flushing of your skin when you ingest alcohol. Sulfonylureas are taken at the same time every day, generally about 30 minutes before a meal. If taken only once a day, they are usually taken with the first meal of the day. Because these medications are broken down by your liver and then eventually leave your body through your urine (via your kidneys), these medications should be used with caution if you have kidney or liver disease. In these diseases, the route by which the medication is broken down or leaves your body may be blocked, which can cause the medicine to accumulate in your body and cause very prolonged hypoglycemia.

Your sulfonylurea is working properly if your blood glucose values remain in a healthy range and you do not suffer from any episodes of hypoglycemia. Check your blood glucose often, both before and after meals, especially if this medication is newly prescribed or your dose has recently been changed. Pay particularly close attention to your glucose readings before your midday and evening meals. Another clue that your medication is working is if your HbA1c is below 7 percent and your blood glucose levels are in a healthy range most of the time. If not, review your activity and eating patterns, ask yourself if you are missing medication doses, and see if there is any pattern to your high or low glucose levels. If your numbers remain too high or too low or you are not satisfied with your control, your doctor may need to change your dose or even switch your medication.

biguanides

Biguanides (bi-gwan-ides) are the second type of diabetes medication. Currently, the only biguanide available in the United States is Glucophage, also known by its generic name, metformin. In the 1960s, a precursor of metformin, DBI-TD (also known as phenformin), was introduced as a twice-a-day medication for the control of glucose levels. It was a very effective medication, but it was removed from the market because of a rare but fatal complication called lactic acidosis. Lactic acidosis is a condition in which lactic acids build up in the bloodstream; it is fatal in 50 percent of the people who develop it. This devastating side effect prompted researchers to develop metformin, a safer version of

DBI-TD. It was introduced in Europe about 40 years ago but was not available in the United States until 1995.

How Glucophage works is not yet completely understood. Its major action is to cause the liver to produce less glucose. Since Glucophage does not directly affect insulin levels and probably does not affect the uptake of glucose by your muscles, it is not very effective for controlling post-meal glucose levels. Its greatest benefit seems to be in decreasing the output of glucose by your liver during periods when you are fasting (such as between meals or at night).

It acts, basically, by disrupting a normal reaction of your liver. In a person without diabetes, both insulin and glucose levels are generally low when it's been more than four hours since the last meal. As a result, the liver normally steps up its own production of glucose in order to keep the brain fed during this period of fasting. Once a meal is eaten, the levels of glucose and insulin in the blood rise, and the liver, sensing the increased insulin, turns down its own production of glucose.

In a person who is insulin resistant, however, the liver doesn't seem to see insulin, even when there is plenty in the bloodstream (such as after a meal), so it doesn't slow its own production; it mistakenly acts as if your blood glucose is low all the time. It continues to make glucose that it releases into your bloodstream—even though, as a person with diabetes, your blood glucose levels are already too high. Glucophage stops this excess glucose production by the liver.

Since the most extended period of fasting for many people occurs overnight, the liver tends to be very busy during that time; as a result, the morning glucose levels tend to be the highest of the day. Glucophage works well to prevent these early-morning highs by decreasing glucose production while you sleep. As an added benefit, it appears to cause less weight gain than most of the other diabetic medications and does not cause hypoglycemia. With all of these positives, it is not surprising that Glucophage is currently the most commonly prescribed diabetic medication in the United States.

These accolades aside, the side effects of Glucophage do mar its sparkling reputation somewhat. About 30 percent of the people who take Glucophage develop stomach upset or diarrhea; about 3 percent of those individuals find these side effects so intolerable that they cannot continue the medication. However, if you start out on a low dose of Glucophage that is slowly increased over time and if you take the medicine with or immediately after a meal, these gastrointestinal side effects can be minimized or eliminated. Sometimes, decreasing the total dose or only taking the medication with the evening meal can eliminate the side effects. If, after trying these adjustments, you are still plagued by diarrhea, loose stools, or frequent or uncontrollable bowel movements, talk to your doctor. Such side effects obviously can decrease your quality of life and you need not tolerate them, since there are other medications available to help you achieve glucose control. A newer version of Glucophage, Glucophage XR, is now available and has fewer gastrointestinal side effects. However, if you take Glucophage XR, be sure to have your triglyceride levels monitored, since this medication may cause them to increase.

Like its predecessor, Glucophage can cause lactic acidosis, but this is extremely rare; only about 30 of every 1 million people who take the drug experience it each year. The signs and symptoms of lactic acidosis are unusual muscle pain, fast and shallow breathing, slow or unsteady heartbeat, vomiting, or a serious infection with dehydration and fever. To avoid this potentially dangerous effect, certain people should not take this medication:

- Glucophage should never be used by anyone who drinks heavily or is a binge drinker. Heavy intake is considered to be more than two to three drinks per day (a drink is 5 ounces of wine, 12 ounces of beer, or 1½ ounces of hard liquor).

- It should not be taken by anyone who has liver disease, such as hepatitis. A test that measures a liver enzyme called *alanine transaminase (ALT)* should be done; elevated levels may indicate that the liver is irritated or diseased.

- It should not be taken by anyone with kidney disease. The creatinine level in your blood is a measurement of your kidney function. For women, this level should be less than 1.4 mg/dl, and for men, less than 1.5 mg/dl. If your creatinine level is too high, you should not take Glucophage.

- In general, Glucophage is not prescribed for people more than 80 years of age unless their kidney and liver functions are tested, frequently monitored, and found to be normal. After age 80, our kidney function naturally decreases. At this age, blood creatinine levels are no longer the best indicator of kidney function. Kidney function is best evaluated by a 24-hour measurement of your creatinine clearance, which requires you to collect your urine for 24 hours straight so that your kidney function can be checked.

- It should not be taken by anyone who has a condition that results in poor circulation, such as congestive heart failure, or a condition that results in a low level of oxygen, such as severe asthma or serious lung disease.

- Caution must also be taken if any type of medical test involving contrast dye is required. During tests that use contrast dye, the kidneys' excretion of lactic acid is slowed, which can allow the acid to build up in the blood. If you need to have such a test, you will need to stop taking Glucophage before the test and not start taking it again for two to three days afterward. You will also need to have your kidney function reevaluated before you restart the medication. However, do not stop taking Glucophage unless and until your doctor has directed you to do so.

Glucophage comes in 500, 850, and 1,000 mg tablets. It is generally taken twice a day, once in the morning and once at night. Occasionally, to minimize side effects, it is taken just once a day, in the evenings, or in smaller doses before each meal, three times a day. The initial dose is usually 500 mg with the evening meal. It is then increased 500 mg each week until the usual maximum dose of 2,000 mg per day is reached. This is generally taken as 1,000 mg, twice a day. Above 2,000 mg per day, there appears to be little added benefit, and additional side effects are likely. If for any reason you must stop taking Glucophage for more than three days, you may find that you have to restart at the 500 mg dose to avoid side effects. Most people who have to stop the medication for just three days to have a contrast-dye study done, however, are able to restart the medication at their usual dose without experiencing significant side effects.

alpha-glucosidase inhibitors

Alpha-glucosidase (glue-kos-a-dase) *inhibitors* are the third type of pill available to treat diabetes. There are two medications available in the United States that fall into this class: Precose (acarbose) and Glyset (miglitol). Both medications work on your small intestines, where starches and large sugar molecules are broken down and absorbed.

One of the primary enzymes that allow for the absorption of glucose into your blood is alpha-glucosidase. This enzyme is in the lining of your small intestines, and its effectiveness is partially blocked by these medications. As a result, glucose is more slowly absorbed, and some glucose may not be absorbed at all but rather digested by bacteria found further downstream in your intestines. This delay in the absorption of glucose into the blood helps to prevent the sudden surges of glucose that can occur after eating. While these medications do not appear to cause weight loss, they cause a moderate lowering of blood glucose after meals and a very mild lowering in the fasting state, such as first thing in the morning.

When alpha-glucosidase inhibitors are used, not all of your food is absorbed, so it has ample time to react with the bacteria and yeast normally found in your bowels. These bacteria and yeast break down starches and sugars into gases. This results in the main side effects reported with these medicines—diarrhea and the tremendous production of gas. About 80 percent of all people who use either one of these medications experience these side effects, and a number of them find they cannot tolerate these effects in the long term. Other side effects are more rare and include liver irritation, so these medications should not be used if you have liver disease. In addition, like Glucophage, the alpha-glucosidase inhibitors can build up in your system if your kidneys are not functioning well. If your creatinine level is or ever exceeds 2.0 mg/dl, you should not take these medications.

Alpha-glucosidase inhibitors cannot cause hypoglycemia by themselves. However, caution is required if they are taken with a medication, such as a sulfonylurea, that can cause low blood glucose levels. Because the alpha-glucosidase inhibitors delay the absorption of certain sugars, hypoglycemia can only be treated with glucose tablets, milk, corn syrup, honey, or fruit juices. The absorption of any other starches or sugars would be delayed, resulting in more prolonged episodes of hypoglycemia.

The usual dose of alpha-glucosidase inhibitors is 25 to 100 mg with each meal, taken no more than three times a day. Any dosage increases should be done *very* slowly, about once every other week or even once a month. This slow increase in dose may lower the potential for side effects and help the body become accustomed to the changes these medications cause.

With their minimal effectiveness and frequent side effects, the class of alpha-glucosidase inhibitors has not been extremely popular with people in the United States who have diabetes. Oddly enough, however, these drugs are the number-one prescribed diabetes medication in Germany.

thiazolidinediones (glitazones)

Thiazolidinediones (thigh-ah-zo-la-deen-die-owns), commonly referred to as

THE CURRENT GLITAZONE LINEUP

BRAND NAME	GENERIC NAME	STRENGTHS	DOSE	MAXIMUM DOSE
Avandia	rosiglitazone	2, 4, and 8 mg	once or twice a day	8 mg
Actos	pioglitazone	15, 30, and 45 mg	once a day	45 mg

glitazones, are the fourth and most controversial group of medications available to treat diabetes. Also known as *TZDs* or *insulin sensitizers,* they ushered in a new age in the treatment of type 2 diabetes when they were first introduced in 1997. For the first time ever, a medication was available to decrease the main problem of type 2 diabetes—insulin resistance.

The glitazones work on the genes inside your fat cells and may work elsewhere in the body as well. They start by stimulating a molecule called *PPAR gamma,* and this stimulation has several results. PPAR gamma causes your fat cells to take up more fatty acids and glucose, leaving fewer fatty acids for your muscle cells. The muscle cells return to using glucose as their preferred fuel source and consequently increase their sensitivity to insulin. This is significant since the muscles normally take up 80 percent of the glucose from a meal.

A similar change occurs in your liver. As your insulin resistance decreases, your liver begins to make less glucose, because it can once again easily "see" the insulin in your bloodstream. Significant changes also happen in the beta cells of your pancreas. First, the drop in glucose and fatty acid levels results in lower insulin levels in your blood. This drop, coupled with what appears to be a direct protective effect that the glitazones have on the beta cells, benefits your beta cells to such an extent that they are able to recover from the stress of diabetes and Syndrome X and live much longer. So the glitazones may actually prevent the downhill slide that eventually leads to the inability of your pancreas to secrete insulin and the subsequent need for insulin injections. And the benefits don't end there.

The glitazones have been shown to have a protective effect on the blood vessels of your body. They reduce the holes in the blood vessels of the kidneys through which albumin is lost, so they may play a direct role in preventing diabetic kidney disease. Studies have also shown that the glitazones improve the condition of your coronary arteries (the blood vessels that feed the heart), not just indirectly by lowering blood fats, but directly. Likewise, when you take

glitazones, your level of beneficial HDL cholesterol increases, your triglyceride level drops, your blood pressure decreases, and your clotting factors improve, all of which decrease your risk of coronary heart disease.

Unfortunately, controversy has surrounded the glitazones since 1999, when Rezulin (troglitazone), the first in this class of medications, made headline news. The news was not good. The early clinical trials of Rezulin had shown that it increases the likelihood of liver irritation threefold. After Rezulin hit the market in 1997, case reports of liver failure and death began to trickle in to the U.S. Food & Drug Administration (FDA). Still, they appeared very rare. At the time, Rezulin was the only glitazone on the market, and more than a million people were successfully managing their diabetes with it. Indeed, it was proving itself to be a very valuable medication. So the FDA agreed that Rezulin could continue to be prescribed but only with more closely monitored liver function testing.

As the liver side effects of Rezulin continued to make news throughout 1999 and early 2000, two new medications in this class hit the market. They were Actos (pioglitazone) and Avandia (rosiglitazone). These two new medications did not appear to cause the serious liver side effects of Rezulin. So the makers of Rezulin stopped making it and removed it from the market in March 2000. Today, literally millions of patients have taken the two new medicines with no evidence of liver complications or side effects any greater than those observed in clinical trials. The new glitazones promise beneficial effects similar to Rezulin, with some minor differences.

Very limited and preliminary studies have suggested differences between Avandia and Actos; these differences can play a role in your doctor's choice of medication for you. Actos appears to be more beneficial in improving lipid levels than Avandia.

So far, the side effects of these drugs appear to be very few. Weight gain, increased risk of hypoglycemia if combined with certain other diabetes drugs, an increased risk of pregnancy, anemia, edema (fluid retention), and liver irritation are possible side effects of both Actos and Avandia.

Why the glitazones cause weight gain is not entirely understood, but it could occur for several reasons. Weight gain is not an uncommon side effect for any medication that improves diabetes control. As your blood glucose levels improve, your body is able to use glucose for energy or save it for future use, instead of losing it in the urine. In other words, your body is now hanging on to the fuel you take in, so if you take in more fuel than you need, your "storage tanks" become that much more visible.

Another common reason for weight gain from diabetes treatment is the food intake required to correct frequent hypoglycemia. Although the glitazones do not cause hypoglycemia when taken alone, combining them with a sulfonylurea, a glitinide, or insulin can result in hypoglycemia. The glitazones decrease your insulin resistance, which allows the other medications to work too well; the result is that you eat more food to keep up with the insulin output that the medications cause. By simply decreasing, or even eliminating, the dose of sulfonylurea, glitinide, or insulin, the frequency of hypoglycemia diminishes, and the weight gain slows. However, you should not significantly decrease your dose or eliminate any medication without prior approval from your diabetes care team.

Some weight gain is caused by fluid retention. The fluid retention is due to a relaxing of your blood vessels, which previously were constricted because of your high insulin levels. This is a good thing for your health, but the extra capacity created by the expansion of your blood vessels ends up getting filled by salt and water. The fluid buildup can lead to edema and can also cause a dilution of your red blood cells, resulting in a mild anemia that is usually nothing to worry about. The edema appears as an increase in your weight, as well as swelling, especially around your feet and ankles. About 5 percent of people who take a glitazone stop taking the medication due to edema. In addition, if you currently have a serious level of congestive heart failure or a history of heart disease, the extra fluid may cause shortness of breath and a worsening of your condition. For these reasons, patients with these conditions who use a glitazone should be monitored closely by their doctor.

An increased risk of pregnancy is also associated with the glitazones. Rezulin, specifically, seemed to make birth control pills less effective in preventing pregnancy. Using an alternative method of birth control generally solves this problem. All medications in this class can increase the risk (or, depending on your viewpoint, improve the chances) of pregnancy as a direct result of their ability to decrease insulin resistance.

Because Avandia and Actos are related to Rezulin, they carry with them the legacy of the Rezulin liver complications. The FDA has required that liver monitoring be done periodically during the first year of glitazone use, even though there have been no reports of liver complications with these newer glitazones.

It takes glitazones longer to become effective in your system than most diabetes medications, which can begin lowering glucose levels within hours of their ingestion. Because the glitazones work on a cellular level, through your genes, the decrease in insulin resistance and subsequent lower glucose levels are very slow to occur. It can take up to four months for you to see the full effect of a glitazone on your glucose levels, but usually you'll notice some improvement within the first one to two weeks. Because of this slow action, your doctor probably won't try increasing your glitazone dose within the first four to six weeks of therapy in order to first see what effect it has had on your blood glucose levels.

glitinides

Glitinides (gli-tin-eyeds) are the fifth and newest type of medication available to treat type 2 diabetes. This class of medications first became available in 1998, with the release of Prandin (repaglinide). Glitinides, which are similar to sulfonylureas, help to lower rising glucose levels by stimulating the beta cells of your pancreas to release insulin. However, they differ from the sulfonylureas in that they are much shorter-acting and begin working very quickly to increase your insulin level while your food is being digested and glucose is entering your bloodstream. In addition to acting quickly, they also leave your bloodstream quickly, so your body doesn't keep releasing insulin beyond when it's needed, thus reducing your risk of hypoglycemia.

Sulfonylureas are generally taken just once a day and cause a steady release of insulin throughout the day, whether you eat or not. Glitinides are different because they are taken just before meals. And because they work very quickly, they allow you to vary the timing and frequency of your meals each day. You take this medication one, two, three, or four times a day, depending on how many meals you eat. If you need or want to miss a meal, you simply skip that pill entirely.

Prandin comes in 0.5, 1, and 2 mg doses. The total daily dose should not exceed 16 mg. Because it prompts your pancreas to release insulin, Prandin has the potential to cause hypoglycemia, especially if you take your pill but your meal is unexpectedly delayed or you eat significantly less than usual. However, the risk of hypoglycemia is less than it is with the sulfonylureas because Prandin is a much shorter-acting medication and therefore does not remain in your system for extended periods after the meal. Other side effects or symptoms that have been reported with Prandin use include cold and flulike symptoms, diarrhea, joint aches, and back pain. In addition, a rash and stomach upset can occur, but they are quite rare.

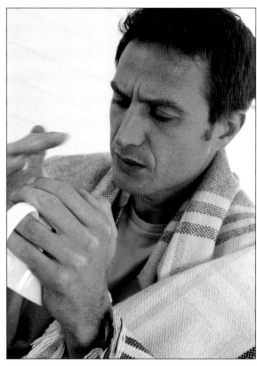

The benefit of the glitinides, when compared to sulfonylureas, is that they do not contain a sulfur group and thus do not cause sulfa allergies. In addition, to date, Prandin is the only medication that can be used safely by people who have kidney and liver problems, as it does not significantly affect these conditions in an adverse way. Still, it must be used with caution and continual monitoring.

Prandin has recently been joined by another glitinide, Starlix (nateglinide). It differs from Prandin in that it is even faster-acting and comes in only two strengths, 60 and 120 mg. Like Prandin, it is taken just before each meal. The benefits of this new medication may include an even lower risk of hypoglycemia.

combination therapy

The new drugs have certainly changed the face of diabetes treatment. Each, alone, helps fix a trouble spot in the diabetes process. But they are increasingly being used in various combinations to make diabetes treatment more individualized—and more successful.

WHERE DO THEY WORK?

TYPE OF MEDICATION	GLITAZONE	BIGUANIDE	ALPHA-GLUCOSIDASE INHIBITOR	GLITINIDE	SULFO-NYLUREA
brand names	Actos Avandia	Glucophage	Precose Glyset	Prandin Starlix	Micronase Diabeta Glynase Glucotrol Amaryl
site of action and metabolic effect	**fat cells** Causes fat cells to take up more fatty acids and glucose, decreasing insulin resistance in the muscles	**liver** Causes liver to produce less glucose	**small intestine** Delays absorption of glucose in small intestine	**pancreas** Stimulates the beta cells to make more insulin	**pancreas** Stimulates the beta cells to make more insulin

meeting more needs

In diabetes, you have multiple problems that need to be fixed, and one pill just can't meet every need. First, your muscles are not taking up the glucose in your bloodstream. Next, your liver is overproducing glucose, further increasing the glucose levels in your blood. And finally, the insulin production by your pancreas cannot keep up with the high levels of glucose in your blood. Different medication types address these various concerns, and sometimes a combination of medications is even more effective in lowering glucose levels than a single medicine.

the one-by-one approach

In the United States, until a few years ago, there was little discussion of using multiple-medication therapy for people with diabetes. The only "combination therapy" was the addition of insulin to the maximum dose of a sulfonylurea, if and when the pills alone could not get the job done. With the release of four new types of medications in the past several years, there are now more than 30 different combinations of medications that can be used to treat diabetes.

The most commonly used method of prescribing medications to improve glucose control is called the "Step System." In this traditional approach, medications are slowly and systematically added, with the goal of achieving glucose control. Because the glitazones address the primary problem in type 2 diabetes, insulin resistance, and because there is no risk of hypoglycemia with these medications, they are considered the best first-line treatment. The next step of glucose control is to add Glucophage, for its additional effect on the liver and, again, because of its lack of hypoglycemia potential. If glucose levels still continue to increase despite the use of these medications, the addition of a sulfonylurea or glitinide may be neces-

How the Possible Combinations Compare

Type of Medication	Biguanide	Alpha-Glucosidase Inhibitor	Glitinide	Sulfonylurea	Insulin
Brand Names	Glucophage	Precose Glyset	Prandin Starlix	Micronase Diabeta Glynase Glucotrol Amaryl	
Glitazone Actos Avandia	Great combination. Lowers glucose output by liver and increases glucose uptake by the muscles. No hypoglycemia.	Slight benefit. Increases glucose uptake by the muscles and improves after-meal glucose levels. No hypoglycemia.	Probably good, but few studies done. Increases glucose uptake by the muscles and stimulates release of insulin at meals. Small risk of hypoglycemia.	Good combination. Increases glucose uptake by the muscles and stimulates release of insulin throughout the day. Risk of hypoglycemia.	Good combination. Glitazone added to insulin allows reduction in insulin dose. Risk of hypoglycemia.
Biguanide Glucophage		Slight benefit. Decreases glucose output by liver and improves after-meal glucose levels. No hypoglycemia.	Probably good, but few studies done. Decreases glucose output by liver and stimulates release of insulin at meals. Small risk of hypoglycemia.	Good combination. Decreases glucose output by liver and stimulates release of insulin throughout day. Risk of hypoglycemia.	Good, but not as beneficial as insulin combined with glitazone.
Alpha-Glucosidase Inhibitor Precose Glyset			Probably good, but few studies done. Stimulates release of insulin at meals and improves after-meal glucose levels. Small risk of hypoglycemia, which must be treated with glucose tabs.	Good combination. Stimulates release of insulin throughout day and improves after-meal glucose levels. Risk of hypoglycemia, which must be treated with glucose tabs.	Possible combination, but no studies done. Improves after-meal glucose levels. Risk of hypoglycemia, which must be treated with glucose tabs.
Glitinide Prandin Starlix				No reason to use both together.	Pills at meals and NPH insulin at bedtime. Stimulates release of insulin at meals and maintains basal insulin needs at night. Risk of hypoglycemia.
Sulfonylurea Micronase Diabeta Glynase Glucotrol Amaryl					Pills during day and NPH insulin at bedtime. Stimulates release of insulin at meals and maintains basal insulin needs at night. Risk of hypoglycemia.

sary. Acarbose (Precose) is occasionally used either prior to or after the addition of a sulfonylurea, but its use in the United States is limited. The final addition to the treatment plan is insulin. The Step System, sometimes also referred to as the "Stutter System," usually fails because it just never seems to catch up to the ever-rising glucose levels. It is a slow approach, and sometimes the doses are not increased quickly enough, which means that glucose levels remain elevated for months before a dose increase or additional medication is tried.

the total overhaul

The reality for most people, when they discover they have diabetes or when they finally decide that they need to take care of themselves, is that their glucose levels are generally quite high. One medication will rarely make the grade. Glucose levels are likely to be in a toxic range, the pancreas can't keep up, and insulin resistance is off the charts. Because everything is so out of control, the "Blast and Taper Fast System" may be a more appropriate method of attack. This approach temporarily forces the pancreas to make more insulin, decreases glucose output by the liver, and addresses the insulin resistance caused by the continuously high glucose levels. With Blast and Taper Fast, a glitazone such as Actos or Avandia is started to decrease insulin resistance, Glucophage is given to decrease the glucose output by the liver, and a sulfonylurea, such as Glucotrol, or a glitinide such as Prandin is used to stimulate the beta cells and increase insulin production. Insulin may even be used early on in this approach. Blood glucose levels are checked frequently (four times per day), and as soon as the glucose levels begin to fall below 120 mg/dl, the insulin and sulfonylurea or glitinide doses are decreased rapidly; they may even be stopped as blood glucose falls into the goal range. As the glitazone takes its full effect, if glucose levels become normal, Glucophage may even be decreased or discontinued as well, as long as the blood glucose remains below 120 mg/dl.

The goal with the Blast and Taper Fast System is to use the maximum dose and number of medications in order to achieve the maximum control as soon as possible. Once glucose levels begin to respond and before hypoglycemia becomes an issue,

COMBINATION MEDICATIONS CURRENTLY AVAILABLE

NAME	COMBINATION	AVAILABLE STRENGTHS
Glucovance	Glyburide and Glucophage	1.25/250, 2.5/500, 5/500
Metaglip	Glipizide and Glucophage	2.5/250, 2.5/500, 5/500
Avandamet	Avandia and Glucophage	1/500, 2/500, 5/500, 2/1,000, 4/1,000

medications are quickly tapered off, starting with any that can cause hypoglycemia, allowing the long-term beneficial effects of the glitazone to continue. In this way, even those people whose diabetes is sorely out of control can begin to improve their condition and lower their risk of complications right away.

fixed combinations

To make diabetes management easier, some drug manufacturers are now making fixed combinations of medications, in which specific doses of two or more drugs are included in a single pill. These combination medications are generally cheaper than buying the individual medications separately and allow you to take a smaller number of actual pills. On the downside, fixed combinations do not allow adjustments to be made to the dosages of the individual medicines.

treatments on the horizon

A promising-looking treatment that is currently being studied is *glucagon-like peptide 1 (GLP-1)*. GLP-1 is a naturally occurring, proteinlike substance found in our intestines. When released, it stimulates the body's insulin secretion, slows the intestinal absorption of glucose, and reduces appetite. In other words, it does exactly what you'd want a treatment for type 2 diabetes to do. Unfortunately, in its current form, it is

broken down in a few minutes. Research into this exciting potential treatment continues and is focused on an oral formula that will prevent this rapid breakdown. Expect to hear more about this in the coming years.

New glitazones are also in the pipeline. Some are more potent, significantly improve lipid levels, and actually cause weight loss. In addition, research involving the newest potential diabetes medications looks extremely promising. These drawing-board medications do not look or act anything like the currently available drugs. But they have a profound effect on cholesterol, lowering it by 80 percent, and they decrease glucose levels, all without any apparent side effects, at least in rats.

Even as things stand, however, the drug treatments available to the person with type 2 diabetes have never been so plentiful—or so effective. The boom in diabetes treatments during the last several years has been so significant that for the first time people can be told that diabetes complications are no longer a given and that achieving absolutely normal blood glucose levels, without hypoglycemia, is an absolute possibility.

using insulin

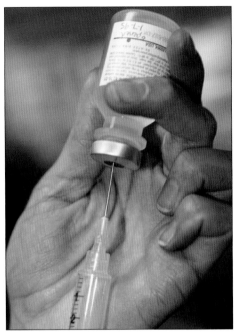

As unpleasant as the thought of having to give yourself a shot might be, it cannot compare to the devastating long-term complications that result from uncontrolled diabetes. Besides, the future of insulin therapy is looking pain free!

sticking to control

Mention the word insulin and just about everyone has a story, and it generally doesn't have a happy ending. "My Aunt Grace started insulin, and shortly afterward she ended up going blind." "I know this guy, he takes insulin and he's always sick." "My friend had to start insulin, and she's gained 40 pounds over the last year!" In addition to personal tales like this, health care professionals have been known to threaten their patients with insulin as a motivational tool. The person is told "If you don't get your act together, take your pills, strictly follow your diet, and start exercising regularly, I'll have to put you on insulin" or "If you fail this, the only thing we have left to try is insulin."

For these reasons, and for the simple fact that very few of us relish the thought of willingly sticking a sharp needle into our skin, insulin has always been viewed as the end of the line, where no other hope exists. This is simply not true. To understand your possible need for insulin, you need to remember the chronic, progressive nature of diabetes. You need to remember that the enemy is not insulin but rather uncontrolled glucose levels. And you need to keep your eye on the ultimate goal: a life lived free of diabetes complications.

As we've said, diabetes is a chronic disease that takes progressively more action to keep glucose levels in a healthy range. You might start out with dietary changes and increased activity as prescribed treatments; then you need a pill; then two pills; then a handful of pills; and finally, a handful of pills and insulin—all to keep your glucose levels within your goal range. Because of the progressive nature of diabetes, if you live long enough, you will need insulin. Some need it sooner than others, and you might need to live to be 137 before you would need it, but given what we know about diabetes today and the treatments we currently have available, you would need insulin eventually.

People often say they'd do anything to get their diabetes under control—anything, that is, but inject insulin. Insulin is viewed by many people with diabetes as signaling the ultimate failure: They've lost control of their diabetes, and there is no hope. They now have the "bad" or "serious" type of diabetes. The reality is that there are only two types of diabetes, the kind that is under control and the kind that isn't, and you want to be in the controlled, uncomplicated group. What you have to do to keep your glucose level under control in no way indicates failure or success, good or bad, serious or not. All diabetes is serious, regardless of what type you have. Commit yourself to doing whatever it takes to keep yourself healthy. Elevated glucose levels result in complications, and if you need to inject insulin to prevent these complications, do it!

the first diabetes treatment

On January 23, 1922, at the University of Toronto, Dr. Frederick Banting and his student C. H. Best made one of the greatest discoveries of the twentieth century. They successfully used insulin to treat a person with diabetes, a

disease that, up to that time, was an automatic death sentence for anyone diagnosed with it. Prior to their discovery, there was no treatment for diabetes. Those with type 1 died very quickly, while those with type 2 died more slowly, suffering horrible complications prior to death. The University of Toronto immediately gave pharmaceutical companies license to produce insulin free of royalties. In early 1923, about a year after the first test injection, insulin became widely available when Eli Lilly and Company marketed Iletin, the first commercially available insulin, which was extracted from the pancreas of stockyard animals.

Animal insulin worked well overall, saving millions of lives, but it was not an exact match with the human hormone and sometimes caused side effects such as skin rashes and allergic reactions that resulted in a loss of tissue at the injection sites. For the next 60 years, insulin would become one of the most studied proteins in the world. During this time, people with diabetes relied on a hormone purified from animals, primarily cattle and pigs.

In 1978, a fledgling biotechnology company named Genentech produced the first synthetically manufactured insulin that could be made in large amounts. Using bacteria or yeast as miniature "factories," the gene for human insulin was inserted into bacterial DNA. The result was human insulin, called *recombinant DNA insulin,* which did not cause the problems that animal insulin sometimes did. When it became widely available in the early 1980s, this new insulin changed the treatment of diabetes forever. Today, almost all people with diabetes who require insulin use a form of recombinant human insulin rather than animal insulin.

one type does not fit all

If you need insulin, the decision to take it is a good one. One thing that we know about insulin is that it always works. It will lower your glucose levels when taken correctly, in the proper amount and at the proper times.

As discussed previously, insulin is a small proteinlike molecule made by the beta cells in the pancreas. Its major actions are to get your muscle and fat cells to take in glucose and to tell your liver to make less glucose. If you have type 1 diabetes, you are *insulin dependent,* as you rely on insulin injections to live. Your pancreas does not make enough insulin, if it makes any at all, to maintain the functions of

your body. If you have type 2 diabetes, you may be *insulin requiring;* you may require insulin to supplement what your pancreas makes in order to maintain the functions of your body.

There are different kinds of insulin, all with different characteristics. When determining the best insulin for you, there are three important characteristics to understand and consider. The first is the *onset* of the insulin. This is the length of time it takes the insulin to reach your bloodstream and begin to lower your glucose level. Next is the *peak time* of the insulin. This is the time when your insulin is at its maximum strength in terms of lowering your glucose level. The last characteristic of insulin to consider is its *duration.* This is the length of time that insulin remains in your body, continuing to work and lower your glucose levels.

With an understanding of these characteristics, you and your diabetes care team have five (soon to be six) different types of insulin to consider. Very often these insulins will be used in some sort of combination in order to meet your required onset, peak-time, and duration-of-action needs. And while the characteristics of insulin types have been studied and documented at length, you need to understand that there is a uniqueness to each of us and that your response to each insulin may vary from what is predicted. For this reason, taking complete, detailed notes of your glucose testing results, the timing of your tests, and your insulin injections becomes vitally important to understanding how insulin works in your body specifically.

the types, your choices

When insulin first became available in 1923, there was only one type, regular insulin. While it was animal-based back then, it is still available today, in a recombinant DNA form. Regular insulin, also called R insulin, is a short-acting insulin that usually begins working within 30 to 60 minutes, peaks two to four hours after injection, and is usually out of your system in six to eight hours.

In the early days of insulin therapy, the needles that were used to inject insulin were thick and needed to be sharpened by hand with a honing stone or razor strap before each use. The syringes were made of glass and needed to be boiled and cleaned every day. The pain and inconvenience of this created a drive to develop an insulin that was longer-acting so that fewer injections were needed. In the 1950s, European researchers developed two new insulin preparations that cut the required four to six injections a day down to two.

The first of these new insulin preparations was NPH insulin, which added a fish protein, protamine, to regular insulin to retard its absorption. NPH is

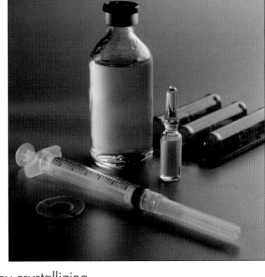

an intermediate-acting insulin that generally starts working in two to four hours, peaks in six to ten hours, and is gone from the system in 16 to 24 hours.

The other new preparation yielded two insulin types, Lente and Ultralente insulin. These insulins were made by crystallizing regular insulin to different degrees. By crystallizing the insulin, it took longer for the insulin to be absorbed, thus prolonging its action in the body. Lente insulin, an intermediate-acting insulin like NPH, generally starts working in three to four hours, peaks in 6 to 12 hours, and lasts for 20 to 26 hours.

By comparison, Ultralente is crystallized to a greater extent and is considered a long-acting insulin. It generally starts working in four to six hours, has its peak action at 10 to 20 hours, and is usually gone from the body 24 to 36 hours after the injection. Because of its extended length of action, it is often referred to as a "peakless" insulin, with a seemingly continuous release over a very long period of time. However, studies have shown that Ultralente insulin is absorbed at different rates in different people. For some people,

Ultralente works like an intermediate-acting insulin, while for other people it is very long-acting.

The newest insulin, released a few years ago, is Lantus, also known as glargine. It is a true "peakless" insulin. This insulin is taken once a day, works consistently for 24 hours, and then is gone. Lantus is rapidly replacing NPH, but because it has a flat, peakless action, Lantus does nothing to lower the glucose rise that results from eating. In addition, because it has a lower pH than other insulins (making it more acidic), it may sting when injected and it cannot be mixed with other insulins in the same syringe.

A fourth type of insulin consists of the rapid-acting insulins Humalog, or insulin lispro, and Novolog, or insulin aspart. This type of insulin begins to work five to ten minutes after it is injected, peaks in about one to two hours, and is gone in about three to five hours. This newer insulin acts much faster than regular insulin and can be injected just prior to a meal, rather than 30 minutes before a meal, which is

ACTIVITY OF THE VARIOUS INSULIN TYPES AVAILABLE TODAY

TYPE OF INSULIN	ONSET	PEAK	DURATION	LOW BLOOD GLUCOSE MOST LIKELY TO OCCUR
rapid-acting lispro, aspart	5–10 minutes	1–2 hours	3–5 hours	2–3 hours
short-acting regular	30–60 minutes	2–4 hours	6–8 hours	3–5 hours
intermediate-acting				
NPH	2–4 hours	6–10 hours	16–24 hours	6–12 hours
Lente	3–4 hours	6–12 hours	20–26 hours	7–14 hours
long-acting				
Ultralente	4–6 hours	10–20 hours	24–36 hours	12–24 hours
Lantus	2 hours	None	13–24 hours	2–24 hours
premixed				
70/30	30–60 minutes	2 & 8 hours	16–24 hours	3 & 9 hours
50/50	30–60 minutes	2 & 8 hours	16–24 hours	3 & 9 hours
75/25 Humalog mix	5–10 minutes	1 & 8 hours	16–24 hours	2 & 9 hours
70/30 Novolog mix	5–10 minutes	1 & 8 hours	16–24 hours	2 & 9 hours

Onset, peak, and duration times are all approximate. Each person is different and will have a unique response to insulin.

recommended for regular insulin. Because it works so fast, it does a better job keeping blood glucose levels down right after eating. Also, because it is cleared from the body so quickly, there is less risk of hypoglycemia. Furthermore, because of Humalog's and Novolog's fast action, there is more flexibility in meal planning and meal timing—a true lifestyle benefit for people who must use insulin.

The final type of insulin is premixed insulin. Premixed insulins consist of different insulins that are combined in fixed percentages. These insulins are convenient for some people who combine two different insulins together, such as NPH and regular. The most typical mixture is 70 percent NPH and 30 percent regular, called 70/30 insulin. Other mixtures that are available are 50/50 insulin, which is 50 percent NPH and 50 percent regular; 75/25 Humalog mix, a combination of 75 percent NPL (a long-acting form of Humalog insulin) and 25 percent Humalog; and 70/30 Novolog mix, a combination of 70 percent NPL and 30 percent Novolog.

Because premixed insulin preparations represent a combination of two different insulins, the onset, peak, and duration of these mixed insulins are a combination of the onset, peak, and duration of each individual insulin. This requires considerably more rigidity in your life, allowing for little variance in

meal timing or amount of food eaten. Premixed insulin is best used by those unwilling or unmotivated to take multiple injections each day, those unable or unwilling to test blood glucose levels frequently, those who have trouble drawing up insulin out of two different bottles, and those without the ability to adjust insulin dosing based on blood glucose readings. You are generally unable to achieve normal glucose control using premixed insulin, and the major goals of this type of rigid insulin therapy are to prevent both low and very high blood glucose levels.

a measure of strength

Pure insulin is a very small, white crystal. When it is made into a solution, it is dissolved or suspended in a liquid. These liquid solutions have different strengths, and the strengths are measured in units of active insulin. The most common insulin available in the United States is U-100 insulin. A U-100 insulin has 100 units of active insulin in each milliliter (mL) of liquid. You can think of it as 100 pieces of insulin in each milliliter of liquid. Using your math skills, this would mean that there are 1,000 units of insulin (10 mL×100 units/mL) in one 10-mL vial of insulin. Other concentrations of insulin, such as U-40, U-50, and U-500 are available, but they are rarely used in the United States today. In Europe and Latin America, U-40 can still be found in use, an important bit of information to know if you are a frequent international traveler.

pick your best shot

Insulin is a protein and therefore cannot be taken orally because the body's digestive juices would destroy it; it must be given by injection. The timing and frequency of insulin injections depend on a number of factors, including the type of insulin, amount and type of food eaten, and the person's level of physical activity. By testing your blood glucose levels frequently and working together with your diabetes care team to analyze your glucose patterns, you and your team will identify the right insulin "fit" for you.

Once your patterns are identified, you then need to choose the insulin delivery system that is right for you. Not too long ago, your only option was a glass syringe with its "sharpen after each use" detachable needle. As metal technology advanced, it was replaced by the disposable needle-and-syringe combination, which had a very sharp, very strong, yet significantly thinner (and thus less painful) needle. Today, syringe needles are so small that in most instances the injection is

almost painless. You often need to look to make sure the needle is through the skin when giving yourself a shot. And when asked, most people who use insulin say that it is a much bigger deal, and more painful, to test your glucose than to administer an injection.

While syringes have greatly improved over the last 75 years, they still require the insulin to be drawn from a vial. This can be inconvenient for anyone attempting to lead a normal, active life, and studies have shown that miscalculated insulin doses are not uncommon. Concerns such as these led to the development of insulin pens, which were first used in Europe and then introduced in the United States in the early 1990s. An insulin pen looks very similar to a fountain pen, except that insulin goes where you would normally find an ink cartridge, and a needle replaces the point of the pen. You "dial up" your desired insulin dose, then you press down on the top to deliver the insulin. Simplifying the process has increased compliance with frequent insulin injections (especially those during the middle of the day, when people are likely to be away from home) and increased the accuracy of the delivered doses. Insulin pens come in two sizes, with 150- or 300-unit cartridges, and in most types of insulin: regular, Humalog, NPH, Premixed 70/30 and 50/50, and 75/25 Humalog Mix.

Despite these advances and the improved compliance they've brought, there are still several bumps in the road to tighter glucose control. The first "bump" is the difficulty in accurately matching the peak-time variability of the intermediate- and long-acting insulins with the rise in glucose levels you have first thing in the morning. This is called the *dawn phenomenon* and is caused by your liver increasing its glucose output every night at about 3:00 A.M. in preparation for the coming day. In order to accurately match your insulin needs, it would be best not to take any long-acting insulin at all but rather to get up at 3:00 A.M. every night to inject regular insulin to correct for this condition. Since that doesn't make for a very good long-term treatment plan, the longer-lasting insulins have been the best alternative.

The second problem occurs when the rate of insulin absorption does not match the glucose rise after meals. This variation can result from the sites you select for injection or the repeated use of a favorite site. For all insulin, except Humalog, Novolog, and Lantus, the insulin absorption rate depends on where you inject it. Insulin injections in the stomach act faster than injections in your arm, injections in your arm act faster than those in your leg, and injections in the buttocks are slowest acting of all. The blood flow to the injection site also governs absorption,

so cold skin makes for slower absorption than does warm skin. Blood flow is also changed when injections are continually given at the same site, because excessive insulin in one area promotes the growth of fat tissue, called *lipohypertrophy*. This fat tissue has few blood vessels and, therefore, absorbs insulin poorly. By changing injection sites (pick a spot about 1 inch from the last injection site), you can generally prevent this problem.

Finally, your daytime, base insulin needs are sometimes difficult to match. Your *base insulin need,* also called your *basal,* is what your body requires to function when you are in a fasting state between meals. The same variation that is associated with the dawn phenomenon occurs in some people in a milder form during the day as well.

To address these problems and to meet the needs of people desiring the best glucose control possible, the late 1970s saw the introduction of the insulin pump, which provided continuous delivery of regular insulin directly under the skin. Unfortunately, the first pumps were not very reliable. By the 1990s, the kinks

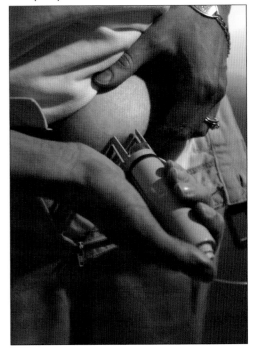

GIVING YOURSELF A SHOT OF INSULIN

WHAT YOU NEED TO DO	WHY YOU NEED TO DO IT
Look at the vial or cartridge of insulin before you use it.	Clumps that do not dissolve, a color change, or cloudiness (of a clear insulin) means the insulin may be damaged and thus no good.
Check the expiration date of the insulin.	Old insulin has lost some of its effectiveness and will not work well or as expected.
If using a normally cloudy insulin, such as NPH or 70/30, gently roll the vial between the palms of your hands. If you are using an insulin pen, invert the pen 15 times to mix the insulin.	Cloudy insulin is a mixture of insulins and/or additives that prolong or change its action. If you don't mix it, you will receive an incorrect percentage of the insulin in this dose as well as in future doses from the same vial.
Wash your hands and clean your injection site.	This prevents infection.
Use a new syringe or new pen needle each time.	This prevents infection. In addition, new needles are sharp. Dull needles hurt.
If using a vial, first draw up air equal to your dose, then inject this air into the vial.	This fills the vial with pressure to help with the withdrawal of the insulin dose.
Turn the vial upside down, and withdraw more than the number of units you need, then push up to the amount you need.	This prevents bubbles in the syringe.
If using an insulin pen, once you attach a new needle to the pen, prime the pen with a 2-unit shot into the air.	This assures that the pen is delivering insulin and fills the needle with insulin in preparation for injecting the proper dose.
Pinch the skin, push the needle straight in, and push the plunger down. Count to 5 before removing the needle. Stop pinching and remove the needle.	This allows for complete delivery of the insulin and prevents insulin leaking back out of the injection site. Congratulations, and well done.

had been addressed and the pumps improved so dramatically that they are currently considered the best method for delivering insulin in almost all people who require insulin. The number of people using pumps in the United States rose from 20,000 in 1995 to more than 80,000 in 1999. This number has been increasing by more than 20,000 new pumpers each year and continues to climb.

The modern pumps are quite similar to the IV (intravenous) machines used in hospitals to deliver medication, only much smaller. They are usually the size of a pager and weigh about four ounces. Each pump has a thin plastic tube, with one end connected to the insulin reservoir inside the pump and the other end to a thin plastic catheter. This catheter is generally placed under the skin of your abdomen using an insertion needle, which is removed once the catheter is in place. The catheter site is changed every two to three days. That means that instead of requiring 8 to 12 insulin injections over the course of two to three days, you need only one needle injection, to place the catheter, during the same time period when you use a pump. Your insulin pump is then programmed to deliver insulin at a specific rate throughout the day and night (your basal rate) to compensate for the dawn phenomenon and meet your daytime base needs. This leaves you free to eat any time, and you are no longer tied to the timing of insulin injections, which significantly reduces the risk of hypoglycemia. Each time you eat, you simply direct the pump to deliver a bolus (or an added amount) of insulin to match the amount of food that you want to eat.

But there are downsides to the pump. One of the major drawbacks is the risk of infection at the insertion site. This is usually remedied by making sure that the site is changed often enough and that a good, clean insertion technique is used. Another and quite serious problem is the very high glucose levels and life-threatening ketoacidosis that can occur if insulin delivery is disrupted for longer than a few hours. This can happen if the pump malfunctions, the tubing becomes kinked or blocked, or the pump runs out of insulin. With all the bells and whistles available on today's pumps, however, a vigilant user is likely to notice such a pump problem before insulin delivery is disrupted for any serious length of time.

The last two hurdles tend to be cost (a pump costs about $6,000) and the issue of constantly being "hooked up" to something. While the cost of a pump is daunting, the cost of keeping an individual with diabetes well is far less than treating someone with complications. Many insurance companies are becoming more aware of this and are beginning to find that the cost of the pump is small compared to the long-term costs of medical care for someone in poor health and poor control. For this reason, with prior authorization, many insurance companies, including Medicare, do cover insulin pumps.

Finally, the concern about being attached to a machine usually fades quickly. Pumps are so small that they are easily slipped into a pocket, clipped onto a belt, or hidden under clothes. Not convinced? Look up pictures of Nicole Johnson, Miss America 1999, wearing her evening gown during the competition. Insulin dependent, she had her pump on during all but the swimsuit portion.

know when to test for ketones

People whose bodies no longer produce insulin and therefore require insulin injections are at risk of developing a serious condition called ketoacidosis. Ketoacidosis can result from high levels of ketones in the blood. If you use insulin, you need to understand what ketoacidosis is, why it happens, how to detect it, and what to do when it occurs.

Ketones are formed when the body doesn't have enough insulin available to allow it to use glucose for energy. Without the required insulin, it simply can't get glucose into its cells. So instead, the body tries to break down stored fat to make fuel available to the cells. The fat in fat cells is broken down into fatty acids, which pass through the liver and form ketones. The ketones begin to build up in the blood; eventually, they spill over into the urine, as well. At high levels, ketones in the blood are toxic and can cause *diabetic ketoacidosis (DKA),* which is a medical emergency.

Ketones can be detected through a simple urine test you can do at home (you can buy the test strips at any pharmacy without a prescription). It is important, however, for you to discuss with your team ahead of time when you should test for ketones and what to do if you detect an elevated level. It is generally recommended that urine be tested for ketones

- when the blood sugar is higher than 240 mg/dl
- during any acute illness (such as pneumonia or severe flu)
- when nausea and/or vomiting are occurring
- during pregnancy (discuss with your team how often)

If you get a urine ketone reading that is above normal, especially if it is accompanied by an elevated blood glucose level, call your doctor at once. And again, be sure you know ahead of time if there are any other situations in which your doctor would like you to test your urine more frequently for ketones.

new directions, new delivery systems

To eliminate the need for insulin injections, various delivery methods have been tried and used, but with limited, if any, success. Mechanical devices, called *jet injectors,* use compressed air to blow the insulin under the skin. They have proven to be expensive, are bulky, and can still be painful, even more so than syringes. Administering insulin through the nose was tried, but without success, because of the irritation that it caused to the mucous membranes of the nose. And the use of rectal insulin suppositories before meals has proved to be socially unacceptable for widespread use.

Holding the most promise is an inhaled spray that is proving to be as effective as injections. These inhaled-insulin delivery systems are currently being tested by at least three manufacturers. With these systems, packages of insulin become airborne in an enclosed cavity and are then inhaled through the mouth. Much to the surprise of many diabetes experts, the inhaled insulin is rapidly absorbed and is not toxic to the lungs. One drawback so far is that the insulin lasts for less than an hour, so it could only be used for mealtime insulin doses. The current systems are also bulky and require a lot of insulin to achieve the same effect as a small injected dose. Still, large studies are underway with hopes of FDA approval sometime in the near future.

Other promising avenues of investigation are the use of ultrasound pulses to deliver insulin through skin patches; implanted, extended-release insulin pellets; and an oral form of insulin. While oral insulin is really a misnomer, researchers have discovered a plant-like substance that can be taken orally and that appears to have effects similar to insulin. Research is underway.

While implantable insulin pumps have been available for years, they are advancing in use quite slowly. A very high insulin concentration (U-400 and higher) is delivered at set bolus (for after meals) and basal (ongoing) rates and is programmed using an external remote control. The pump needs to be refilled about every three months and, until recently, was plagued by incidents of blockage in the delivery catheter. Reformulations of the insulin being delivered through these pumps seem to have improved the blockage situation. By combining this implantable pump with an implantable glucose sensor, the diabetes loop would be closed, creating a "mechanical" cure for diabetes. Such a system may become a reality sometime in the near future.

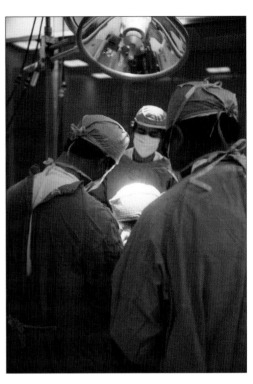

Meanwhile, Canadian scientists made an exciting breakthrough in islet cell transplant research. They have demonstrated a possible cure for type 1 diabetes, with people remaining insulin independent, with normal glucose levels, without significant side effects or complications. This research has lead to worldwide trials, using what is now called the Edmonton Protocol. This, coupled with discoveries by California researchers who have been able to grow beta cells, resulting in an unlimited source of transplant material, may foretell an end to insulin-dependent diabetes.

Even though insulin is not a cure for diabetes, the 1922 medical discovery saved, and continues to save, millions of lives around the world. And while this Nobel Prize winning accomplishment is among one of the greatest medical achievements ever, outside of Sir Frederick G. Banting Square at the Banting Museum in London, Ontario, the Flame of Hope still burns. Only when a cure, rather than a treatment, for diabetes is found, will the flame be extinguished.

fighting hypoglycemia

Diabetes management focuses on lowering high blood glucose, but there's an opposite effect called a hypoglycemic reaction that can be equally dangerous. Especially for people who have had diabetes for a long time or who take medication or insulin, being able to recognize and treat hypoglycemia is a basic skill for their diabetes tool kit.

strange happenings

It's 5:00 P.M.: You test your blood glucose and take your diabetes medication. You start to eat your dinner but, midway through, the phone rings, taking you away from the meal. By the time you return, the food is cold and

you decide not to finish what's left on your plate. All is fine until a few hours later, when you start to feel dizzy and nauseated, begin sweating, and notice that your heart is beating very fast and hard. You test your blood glu-

cose—the meter reads 52 mg/dl! You grab some orange juice, a few cookies, and a handful of grapes. You start feeling a bit better, and by the time you finish a glass of milk and a turkey sandwich, you're on solid ground and everything is back to normal. You check your glucose again before heading to bed and are shocked to find a reading of 269 mg/dl. What the heck is going on?

In two words, you experienced a *hypoglycemic reaction.* The high blood glucose level that followed, called a *food rebound,* resulted from the lifesaving steps you took to increase your blood glucose.

what is hypoglycemia?

As its name suggests, hypoglycemia means low blood sugar (*hypo* means low and *glycemia* means sugar). It's sometimes referred to as an "insulin reaction," "a low," "insulin shock," or just plain "shock." No matter the term used, hypoglycemia is one of the most common, and most dangerous, side effects of any medication for lowering blood glucose.

For the person with diabetes, the goal of treatment is to lower blood glucose levels to as close to normal as possible. If the treatment plan to obtain this goal includes insulin and/or one of the insulin-stimulating medications (a sulfonylurea or glitinide), then hypoglycemia is definitely a risk. Hypoglycemia can occur if you take too much insulin or too large a dose of medication, miss or delay a meal, eat too little food for the amount of insulin or pills taken, increase your normal level of activity, drink alcohol, or any combination of these factors.

As stated previously, the normal range for blood glucose is 70 to 99 mg/dl (measured on a plasma-calibrated meter). If your blood glucose falls below this level, you're in trouble. Your brain and nervous system, remember, depend solely on glucose for energy. In an attempt to raise the glucose level, your brain sends out emer-

gency signals. As a result, your alpha cells, located in your pancreas, release glucagon. The glucagon signals your liver and muscles to release stored glycogen and change it back to glucose to try to raise your blood glucose level to a normal range. Meanwhile, the release of the hormone epinephrine increases your hunger and causes a resistance to insulin's action. Other hormones, cortisol and growth hormone, are also released to counteract insulin and raise your blood glucose levels.

Outwardly, you may begin to feel dizzy, hungry, sick to your stomach, shaky, or very fatigued and weak. You may notice that you are sweaty, your

SYMPTOMS OF HYPOGLYCEMIA

EARLY SYMPTOMS CAUSED BY THE RELEASE OF EPINEPHRINE AND DECREASING BLOOD GLUCOSE LEVELS	LATER SYMPTOMS CAUSED BY THE DECREASING AVAILABILITY OF GLUCOSE TO YOUR BRAIN
Dizziness	Headache
Pale or flushed face	Blurred vision
Irritability	Slurred speech
Hunger	Confusion
Sweating	Euphoria
Rapid heartbeat	Hostility
Fatigue or weakness	Lack of coordination
Nervousness or anxiousness	Drowsiness
Shakiness	Convulsions
Queasiness	Loss of consciousness

How to treat a low blood glucose level

1. Check your blood glucose, if you are able.

2. If you are in doubt and unable to check your blood glucose, ALWAYS assume that your glucose level is low.

3. Eat 15 grams of a fast-acting carbohydrate. That's equal to any of the following:
   3–4 glucose tabs
   4 ounces of fruit juice
   5 sugar cubes
   1 small box of raisins
   1 cup of skim milk
   1 tablespoon of honey
   6 hard candies

4. Wait 15 minutes, then check your blood glucose level again.

5. If symptoms are still present or blood sugar is less than 70, repeat step 3.

6. **If the person is unable to swallow or becomes unconscious, a glucagon injection must be given immediately!** This should be done even if you are unsure that the person's blood sugar is low.

7. If symptoms are gone and it is more than one hour from a mealtime, eat a small snack that includes protein, fat, and carbohydrate, such as a turkey sandwich with mayonnaise.

8. Call your doctor if you experience frequent or severe hypoglycemic reactions.

heart is beating fast, your face is pale or flushed, or your mouth and lips are tingling or numb. These early signs of low blood glucose are primarily caused by the release of epinephrine.

If the glucose continues to drop, less and less is available to your brain. You may develop a headache, blurred vision, slurred speech, and confusion. You may become quite uncoordinated, and your general state of mind may be either euphoric or quite hostile and belligerent. If the low glucose level continues, you may lose consciousness, have a seizure, and possibly lapse into a coma. Hypoglycemia can even result in death.

how do I treat it?

The best time to treat hypoglycemia is as soon as you recognize the first symptoms. Do not wait! Food is the best remedy for hypoglycemia, but not just any food. You want something that will get into your system fast and raise your glucose levels quickly.

While a chocolate bar may seem like a wonderful choice, it actually takes quite a bit of time for it to raise your blood glucose levels. The sucrose from the granulated sugar in the candy bar starts the process, but the fat in the chocolate actually delays the rise in your blood glucose.

Instead, you want something that will get into your system quickly, something that works immediately to raise your blood glucose levels. Simple carbohydrates and liquid carbohydrates are your best choices in this regard. Glucose tablets, sugar cubes, fruit juice, milk, and hard candies are your best bets. They are absorbed quickly into your bloodstream and begin raising blood glucose levels within five to ten minutes of ingestion.

Untreated hypoglycemia or a delay in treating a low blood glucose level can result in a severe hypoglycemic reaction in which you are unable to swallow liquids or food and may even become unconscious. Anyone who takes insulin to manage their diabetes is most at risk for this type of reaction. Others at risk for severe hypoglycemia are those who have had diabetes for many years and have developed something called hypoglycemia unawareness, in which they have difficulty recognizing the symptoms of low blood sugar until it is too late and they are unable to help themselves.

For anyone who takes insulin and anyone with hypoglycemia unawareness, an additional safety net, a glucagon emergency kit, needs to be kept on hand for emergencies. The glucagon in the kit can be given by injection to the person having the severe hypoglycemic reaction. This injected glucagon is a synthetic version of the hormone found naturally in the alpha cells of the pancreas, the hormone that signals the liver and muscles to release stored glycogen. Anyone who is at risk for severe hypoglycemia

should have a glucagon emergency kit and needs to train those around them how to use it. The kit is available, with a doctor's prescription, at pharmacies. Be sure to have the pharmacist or your diabetes care team demonstrate the use of the kit to you so that you can show others how to use it.

prepare yourself and others

If you take insulin or an insulin-stimulating medication, you can reduce your risk of hypoglycemia. It's all a matter of education and preparation. Check your blood glucose levels frequently. Anticipate situations that may trigger hypoglycemia and take steps to adjust; plan ahead for increased activity or changes in routine. Learn how to recognize and treat symptoms of low blood glucose, and stash sugar *everywhere.* Wear identification that states you have diabetes. Teach friends and family how to recognize symptoms of low blood glucose and how to help if you hit a low. And if you take insulin, make sure those around you know how to treat you in case you become disoriented or unconscious and know where you keep your glucagon emergency kit.

expand your options, improve your choices

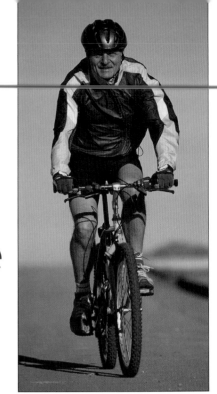

There's no question your food choices and eating habits can have a major impact on your diabetes control. And because you have diabetes, you may assume you must follow a very strict diet. The problem is, diets tend to be seen as temporary. They can also be boring, inconvenient, even frustrating. And, if they cut out foods you truly enjoy, they can lead to problem eating habits such as bingeing. If instead you expand your food options and learn to make healthier food choices that match your tastes and your body's needs for carbohydrate, fat, and other nutrients, you build a skill that will last a lifetime. And that skill can help you control not only your glucose levels, but your blood pressure, cholesterol level, and weight, as well.

learning to choose

Many of us know what it's like to be on a diet, whether it's for our weight, blood pressure, cholesterol, or diabetes. We're quick with the phrase, "I can't, I'm on a diet." That's what dieting is about after all. Not being able to eat all the foods we enjoy. Most often, the foods we *are* allowed are bland or boring. We'd give up anything to have something sweet or rich or flavorful. Eventually, we give up the diet instead. We go back to old habits—or develop new ones, like bingeing—that leave us back where we started—or worse off.

It's unfortunate, too, since how and what we eat and how we live can go a long way toward helping us improve our blood pressure, cholesterol levels, and glucose control, as well as shed some unwanted pounds— all of those Syndrome X problems that people with diabetes struggle with. There is a better way. It's a path that in many ways is the opposite of dieting. It's called learning to choose. It's a path you can stay on for life. It's a skill that can bring the joy and pleasure back into eating as it tackles diabetes, Syndrome X, and heart disease. Unlike dieting, which is all about restrictions, learning to choose healthier foods and eating habits is about expanding your dietary horizons. Here's some advice on learning to choose:

know how foods affect your body. As discussed in Eating for Better Control, you need to check your glucose after meals to find out how different levels of carbohydrates affect your blood glucose. And in the pages that follow, you'll learn how various types of fat affect blood cholesterol and how salt affects blood pressures. Use this information, along with the Nutrient Counter and food labels, to compare foods and make healthier choices.

never call a food good or bad. No single food, in and of itself, is good or bad. A chocolate bar, an ice cream sundae, a piece of prime rib, a slice of bread—not one of these is bad, despite what you may have heard. Nor does eating one of these mean you've failed somehow. Even though you have diabetes, each food can fit into your healthy eating plan, as long as you adjust for it. Likewise, having one of these foods will not make or break your efforts at lowering your cholesterol or losing weight. It won't erase progress you've already made. And if enjoying it once in a while, in a reasonable portion, keeps you satisfied and out of the denial-binge trap, then it helps you in the end.

expand your food options. Go ahead, dive into those grocery aisles and start experimenting! Use the Nutrient Counter and recipes in this book. The more foods you try, the more likely you are to find a wide variety of tasty, desirable foods that match your body's nutrient needs and move you closer to your health goals. Again, it doesn't mean you can't have your old favorites once in a while. But when you want something chewy or creamy or crunchy, you'll also have some options that are lower in calories, fat, or sodium.

say no to quick—or temporary—fixes. When you go on a diet, you generally pick a date to begin (and binge on all your favorites the night before). And when you start, there's often an assumption that you will reach a certain goal—or give up—and go off the diet. Learning to choose isn't like that. It's more like learning how to ride a bike. It may take a while to get the hang of it, but once you learn how, you don't really ever forget. Each time you eat becomes an opportunity to

choose something lower in salt or fat, something higher in fiber, a carbohydrate that's richer in vitamins, or a lower-calorie food or snack. You make the changes as you are able. Eventually, making healthier choices becomes the norm, so there's no reason to fret about an occasional sloppy burger or scoop of double-fudge ice cream. What's more, along the way, you discover you've actually dropped a few pounds, improved your control, and lowered your blood pressure and cholesterol.

By learning to choose rather than trying yet another diet, the ball is in your court. It is up to you how often you make a healthier food choice, how quickly you move toward your goals, and exactly what a healthy, enjoyable diet consists of *for you*. It can seem daunting at first. With freedom comes responsibility. There's nobody telling you what you can and can't eat every day. But once you begin to expand your food choices and discover how truly flavorful even healthier foods can be, you'll realize why learning to choose is such a great choice.

opting for less salt

Relieving the pressure

In addition to limiting sodium, there are other dietary factors that play a role in controlling high blood pressure. In general, high blood pressure can be lowered with a diet that is:
- low in saturated fat, cholesterol, total fat, red meat, and simple carbohydrates
- rich in fruits, vegetables, low-fat dairy foods, whole-grain products, fish, poultry, and nuts

Blood pressure is also helped by a diet that is rich in magnesium (widely available; nuts, seeds, dried beans, and bananas are rich sources), potassium (fruits and vegetables), and calcium (dairy products), as well as protein and fiber.

Sodium, a component of salt, is an essential mineral for the human body. It controls fluid balance, and too little of it can cause serious problems. For some people, however, too much sodium contributes to high blood pressure, which increases the risk of heart attack, stroke, and kidney problems. High blood pressure, as we've said, is especially common in, and dangerous for, people with type 2 diabetes. So it just makes sense, as you're learning to choose more foods—and more healthier foods—to keep an eye out for sodium content and tilt your food choices toward lower-sodium options.

So how much sodium do you need, and how much is too much? The minimum sodium requirement, under normal conditions, is 400 milligrams (mg) a day. That may sound like a lot, until you realize that equals about one-fifth of a teaspoon of table salt. The maximum recommended level is currently 2,400 mg, although new recommendations are pending that will probably lower this level to 1,500 mg a day. Keep in mind, too, that these minimums and maximums include not only salt you sprinkle on your food, but also the salt used in cooking, preparing,

and/or processing the food. And you'd be surprised at the amount of sodium there is in most processed foods (see "Sodium Surprises").

Processed foods account for most of the salt and sodium consumed, so it's important to read food labels (or check the Nutrient Counter in this book) to see just how much sodium foods contain. A good rule of thumb when it comes to sodium is that if the food comes in a bag, in a box, in a can, out a window (of a fast-food joint), or on a restaurant platter, it probably has more sodium than you expect or want (unless you've specifically chosen a lower-salt version).

Here are some additional tips to help you lower your sodium intake:
- Choose reduced-sodium or no-salt-added products.
- Buy fresh. There's no salt added to fresh produce.
- Use fresh poultry, fish, and lean meats more often than canned, smoked, or processed types.
- If you're a fan of soy sauce or teriyaki sauce, try a low-sodium version.
- Experiment with spices. Try fresh herbs in cooking, in salsa and dips,

and in salads. Make your own blend of favorite herbs and spices. You might even consider growing a miniature herb garden on your kitchen windowsill so you'll have fresh herbs at hand year round.

- Go for brown rice, whole-grain pasta, and whole-grain hot cereals cooked without salt.

- If you like tuna, buy water-packed and rinse the meat to remove some of the salt.

- Take the salt shaker off the table. Always taste your food before adding any salt.

- Choose only small portions of foods that are pickled, cured, in broth, or bathed in soy sauce, since these will have higher sodium contents.

- When dining out, ask that your food be prepared without added salt, monosodium glutamate (MSG), or high-sodium ingredients. If they won't accommodate your request, choose another restaurant next time.

- Try limiting salty condiments such as ketchup, mustard, pickles, and may-onnaise. Experiment: Try at least one bite of your food without condiments. If you still miss them, add on just enough to get a hint of their taste, but not so much that you hide the flavor of the food itself. If you don't like the taste of the food without the condiments, choose a different food next time—one whose unadorned flavor you do enjoy.

SODIUM SURPRISES

MINIMAL SODIUM	LOW SODIUM	MODERATE SODIUM	HIGH SODIUM
apple, 1 = 2 mg	applesauce, 1 cup = 6 mg	apple pie, ⅛ pie = 200 mg	apple turnover, 1 fast-food = 400 mg
low-sodium bread, 1 slice = 8 mg	white bread, 1 slice = 114 mg	pound cake, 1 slice = 170 mg	English muffin, 1 whole = 200 mg
olive oil, 1 tbsp = 0 mg	unsalted butter, 1 tbsp = 2 mg	butter, salted, 1 tbsp = 116 mg	margarine, 1 tbsp = 140 mg
fresh corn, 1 ear = 1 mg	frozen corn, 1 cup = 7 mg	corn flakes, 1 cup = 256 mg	canned corn, 1 cup = 384 mg
cucumber, 7 slices = 2 mg	sweet pickle, 1 = 128 mg	cucumber w/ salad dressing = 234 mg	dill pickle, 1 = 928 mg
lemon, 1 = 1 mg	catsup, 1 tbsp = 156 mg	soy sauce, 1 tbsp = 1,029 mg	salt, 1 tbsp = 1,938 mg
potato, 1 = 5 mg	potato chips, 10 chips = 200 mg	mashed potatoes, instant, 1 cup = 485 mg	potato salad, ½ cup = 625 mg
tuna, fresh, 3 oz = 50 mg	tuna, canned, 3 oz = 384 mg	tuna pot pie, 1 frozen = 715 mg	fish sandwich, 1 fast-food = 882 mg
peanuts, unsalted, 1 cup = 8 mg	peanut butter, 1 tbsp = 81 mg	peanut brittle, 1 oz = 145 mg	dry roasted peanuts, salted, 1 cup = 986 mg

falling for less fat

More for less!

Eating less fat can do more than help lower your blood cholesterol and keep your heart and blood vessels healthy. Eating less fat can also help you control your weight, since fat packs more than twice the calories of protein or carbohydrate. And, as previously discussed, because fat can indirectly elevate blood glucose levels by blocking the action of insulin, eating less fat can help improve your blood glucose control.

The connection may not seem obvious, but if you have diabetes, you need to be concerned about your heart. People with diabetes are three times more likely to develop heart disease. One factor contributing to that increased risk is the high blood cholesterol common among people with type 2 diabetes (it's one of the Syndrome X conditions). So as you learn to choose healthier foods, it's important to keep your blood cholesterol level and your risk of heart disease in mind—and in check. To do so, research suggests you choose a diet in which less than 30 percent of calories comes from fat, and of that fat, very little comes from saturated and trans fats.

That's not to say fat is bad, of course. Fat provides energy, and we need some fat to absorb the fat-soluble vitamins A, D, E, and K. And no one can deny fat adds flavor and juiciness to food. It's just that we tend to eat more of it than our bodies can handle in a healthy manner. And because we are inundated with processed foods, we tend to choose foods higher in the fats that can raise our cholesterol and damage our arteries.

To improve our fat choices, then, we need to understand our fat options.

There are three main types of fats: saturated, monounsaturated, and polyunsaturated. The more saturated a fat is, the more detrimental it can be when eaten in excess. Too much saturated fat leads to more of those nasty little LDL molecules, the "bad" cholesterol that lingers in the bloodstream and makes damaging cholesterol deposits in our arteries. Monounsaturated fats have the opposite effect, lowering the number of LDL molecules. As for polyunsaturated fats, their effect depends on their type. One type, called *omega 6 fatty acids*, when eaten in large amounts, can cause water retention, raise blood pressure, increase blood clotting, and decrease "good" HDL cholesterol. The other type, *omega 3 fatty acids*, tends to lower blood cholesterol and heart disease risk by making blood less likely to clot. As for trans fats, they're created when unsaturated fats are "resaturated," making them more solid and increasing their shelf life but also making them act more like saturated fats in the body; they tend to raise total blood cholesterol.

While this may sound a bit complicated, it boils down to choosing more foods that have less total fat and substituting healthier fats for some of the saturated ones you usually eat. Here's some advice to guide you:

- Use the Nutrient Counter in this book and the labels on foods to help you opt more often for foods that have less total fat and less saturated fat.
- Spend more of your choices on a variety of fruits and vegetables, whole-grain products, beans, and nuts. Fruits and vegetables are naturally low in fat (if you don't slather them with fatty sauces) and provide loads of nutrients. Whole-grain foods and beans are low in fat but are nutrient dense and pack a load of fiber, which can fill you up on fewer calories. And nuts, while not especially low in fat, are filled with mostly monounsaturated fats.
- Choose fish (its fat is mostly monounsaturated) more often than poultry (its fat is more saturated), and choose poultry (lower in saturated fat and usually lower in total fat) more often than meat (higher in saturated fats).
- Trim visible fat (it's saturated) from meat and fat and skin from poultry before eating. Instead of frying, which requires added fat, try baking, broiling, roasting, or grilling.
- Include fat-free and low-fat milk products.
- Choose fats and oils that are trans-fat free and have two grams or less saturated fat per tablespoon, such as liquid and tub margarine, canola oil, and olive oil. (Try dipping fresh, crusty bread into olive oil instead of slathering it with butter.)

WHERE ARE THEY?

Saturated fats	Red meat, poultry, cheese, butter, and full-fat dairy products; some plant products, such as palm, coconut, and palm kernel oils
Monounsaturated fats	Olive, canola, and peanut oils; olives; avocados; most nuts, including almonds, cashews, pecans, and pistachios; and peanuts and natural peanut butter
Polyunsaturated fats	**Omega 6s:** Corn, sunflower, soybean, and cottonseed oils; MANY processed foods **Omega 3s:** Many fish, including wild salmon, mackerel, sardines, herring, anchovies, rainbow trout, bluefish, caviar, white albacore tuna; canola oil; flaxseed and flaxseed oil; walnuts and walnut oil; and dark green, leafy vegetables
Trans fats	Many breads, crackers, cookies, doughnuts, frozen pie crusts, deep-fried foods, foods with chocolate coatings, fast foods, packaged and convenience foods, snack items such as chips, cake mixes, pastries, whipped toppings, nondairy creamers, shortening, and some margarines

weighing the benefits

By now you probably realize (or your doctor has told you) that being overweight—especially carrying too much fat in your abdominal area—hampers diabetes control. So you may be wondering where you'll find the weight-loss diet in this book.

Well, you won't. It's not that we think weight loss is unimportant—far from it. It's just that a restrictive diet is not the best way to achieve the benefits of weight loss. For people with diabetes, the best path to weight loss is the same one that leads to getting well and staying well. It's the one you take each time you choose a healthier food or more physical activity. That's right! Rather than deprive yourself to achieve some ideal body size, you simply focus on making one simple choice at a time that will help you control your glucose, blood pressure, and cholesterol. Along the way, you leave an excess pound here, a little excess risk there, and you end up feeling better and more in control.

losing weight does help

There's no denying weight loss is beneficial for people with type 2 diabetes who are overweight. But you don't need to lose 50 or 100 pounds to reap the benefits. Even a weight loss of just 5 to 10 percent of your total body weight can bring impressive improvements in your health. For a person who weighs 200 pounds, that's a weight loss of as little as ten pounds!

Studies show that when a person who has recently been diagnosed with diabetes loses weight, blood glucose levels drop, blood pressure improves, and cholesterol levels return to a healthier range. Medications may be decreased or even stopped altogether.

For a person with long-standing diabetes (of more than 8 to 12 years), weight loss causes the same improvements in glucose, blood pressure, and cholesterol, which can improve well-being and help delay complications. However, losing weight is no longer likely to mean less medication or a delay in the need for insulin. That's because diabetes is a progressive disease, and, despite weight loss, over time the beta cells of the pancreas gradually fail. This is not a failure of the person or of the lifestyle changes; it's the sad nature of a progressive disease.

so why not diet?

The reasons are many. An important one is that you're not trying to lose pounds to look better at a reunion or fit into swimwear. It's your health on the line. And when being healthier is your goal, it makes no sense to use unhealthy habits, like restricting foods or food groups, skipping meals, or depriving yourself of needed energy or nutrients, to reach it.

Besides, it's possible to be slimmer and still have the poor eating habits and inactive lifestyle that cause problems with glucose control, high blood pressure, and high blood cholesterol.

And diets simply don't work in the long run. Within two years of going off a diet, 70 percent of dieters will regain at least half their lost weight, and the five-year success rate of any diet is a measly 3 percent.

what does work?

Basically, the same changes you need to make to improve your glucose control, including an overall diet that gets less than 30 percent of its calories from fat, but here are a few more tips:

fill up on fiber. Foods that are high in fiber can help you feel fuller longer on fewer calories and without increasing your blood sugar.

think small. Choose smaller, more reasonable portions of everything, served on smaller plates (never eat directly from a bag or box or while standing at the kitchen counter), and eat more slowly so you'll "hear it" when your stomach tells you you're full.

check your thirst. Many people confuse feelings of thirst for hunger. So enjoy a large glass of ice water, hot tea, low-sodium broth, or another calorie-free beverage before reaching for food. You may discover that you were really just thirsty.

make trades. When you opt for a food or meal that's fat rich and/or calorie dense, choose other foods and meals that day that are low in fat and light in calories.

add even more activity. The more you move, the more you'll lose. We've pointed out that physical activity is an essential element in controlling diabetes. But every extra bit of planned exercise and even unplanned activity (running errands, taking stairs instead of elevators, parking farther from stores, etc.) helps burn calories.

the nutrient counter

To help you learn and track how individual foods affect your blood sugar levels, we've included this nutrient counter, which lists the carbohydrate content of hundreds of foods. It also provides information on nutrients such as calories, fat, cholesterol, and sodium to aid you in managing other medical conditions, including high blood pressure, high blood cholesterol, and excess weight, that often accompany diabetes. The counter can assist you as you begin to explore all the food options out there, measure and record how each new food affects your glucose levels, and make choices that improve your diabetes control. Don't feel you must choose only items listed here, though. Use this listing as a starting point and handy reference, then hit the grocery aisles, using food labels for items not listed here.

Remember, it's variety you're after. By paying attention to how a specific food affects your glucose, watching portion sizes, and mixing and matching foods with varying amounts of carbs, you can fit just about any food or dish into your diabetic meal plan.

For each food item, the counter lists a specific portion size. (If the portion you eat is twice as large as the amount stated, don't forget to double the calorie, carb, and other nutrient values!) For the specified portion of each food item, the counter lists the calories; the grams of total carbohydrate (that's the simple and complex carbs as well as the fiber), fiber (you can subtract this amount from the total carbs to get the amount of usable, or digestible, carbs), total fat, saturated fat, and protein; and the milligrams of cholesterol and sodium. Values have been rounded to the nearest whole number. If "Tr" (which stands for trace) appears in a column, it means there's less than half a gram of that nutrient. If "na" appears, that means the value was not available to us. Every effort was made to ensure that the information shown here was accurate at the time of printing.

The counter information itself was adapted from the Nutrient Database for Standard Reference, Release 16–1 (2004), from the Agricultural Research Service of the U.S. Department of Agriculture. To access the home page of the Nutrient Data Laboratory, type www.nal.usda.gov/fnic/foodcomp into your Internet browser.

FOOD, PORTION	CALORIES	TOTAL CARB (G)	FIBER (G)	TOTAL FAT (G)	SAT FAT (G)	CHOL (MG)	PROTEIN (G)	SODIUM (MG)
BAKED PRODUCTS								
Bagel, cinnamon-raisin, 3½" dia	195	39	2	1	Tr	0	7	229
Bagel, egg, 3½" dia	292	56	2	2	Tr	25	11	530
Bagel, plain (includes onion, poppy, sesame), 3½" dia	289	56	2	2	Tr	0	11	561
Biscuit, mixed-grain, refrigerated dough, 2½" dia	116	21	na	2	1	0	3	295
Biscuit, plain or buttermilk, commercially baked, 2½" dia	127	17	Tr	6	1	Tr	2	368
Bread, cornbread, dry mix, prepared, 1 piece	188	29	1	6	2	37	4	467
Bread, cracked-wheat, 1 slice	65	12	1	1	Tr	0	2	135
Bread crumbs, grated, seasoned, 1 oz	104	20	1	1	Tr	Tr	4	751
Bread, French or Vienna (includes sourdough), 4"×2½"×1¾"	175	33	2	2	Tr	0	6	390
Bread, Italian, 1 slice	54	10	1	1	Tr	0	2	117
Bread, mixed-grain (includes whole-grain, 7-grain), 1 slice	65	12	2	1	Tr	0	3	127
Bread, raisin, 1 slice	71	14	1	1	Tr	0	2	101
Bread, rye, 1 slice	83	15	2	1	Tr	0	3	211
Bread stick, plain, 7⅝"×⅝"	41	7	Tr	1	Tr	0	1	66
Bread stuffing, dry mix, 6 oz package	656	130	5	6	1	2	19	2703
Bread, wheat (includes wheat berry), 1 slice	65	12	1	1	Tr	0	2	133
Bread, wheat, reduced-calorie, 1 slice	46	10	3	1	Tr	0	2	118
Bread, white, 1 slice	67	13	1	1	Tr	0	2	170
Bread, whole-wheat, 1 slice	69	13	2	1	Tr	0	3	148
Cake, angelfood, 1/12 of 12 oz cake	72	16	Tr	Tr	Tr	0	2	210
Cake, chocolate, with chocolate frosting, ⅛ of 18 oz cake	235	35	2	10	3	27	3	214

Food, portion	Calories	Total Carb (g)	Fiber (g)	Total Fat (g)	Sat Fat (g)	Chol (mg)	Protein (g)	Sodium (mg)
BAKED PRODUCTS (CONT.)								
Cake, pound, 1/10 of cake	116	15	Tr	6	3	66	2	119
Cake, shortcake, biscuit-type, prepared from recipe, 1 oz	98	14	na	4	1	1	2	143
Cake, white, prepared from recipe, no frosting, 1/12 of 9" dia cake	264	42	1	9	2	1	4	242
Cheesecake, 1/6 of 17 oz cake	257	20	Tr	18	8	44	4	166
Coffeecake, fruit, 1/8 cake	156	26	1	5	1	4	3	193
Cookie, chocolate sandwich, with creme filling, 1 cookie	47	7	Tr	2	Tr	0	Tr	60
Cookies, animal crackers, 2 oz box	254	42	1	8	2	0	4	224
Cookies, butter, 1 cookie	23	3	Tr	1	1	6	Tr	18
Cookies, chocolate chip, soft-type, 1 cookie	69	9	Tr	4	1	0	1	49
Cookies, fig bars, 1 cookie	56	11	1	1	Tr	0	1	56
Cookies, fortune, 1 cookie	30	7	Tr	Tr	Tr	Tr	Tr	22
Cookies, oatmeal, 1 oz	128	19	1	5	1	0	2	109
Cookies, peanut butter, 1 cookie	72	9	Tr	4	1	Tr	1	62
Cookies, raisin, soft-type, 1 cookie	60	10	Tr	2	1	Tr	1	51
Cookies, sugar (includes vanilla), 1 cookie	72	10	Tr	3	1	8	1	54
Crackers, cheese, 1 cracker, 1" sq	5	1	Tr	Tr	Tr	Tr	Tr	10
Crackers, cheese, sandwich-type with peanut butter filling, 1 sandwich	32	4	Tr	2	Tr	0	1	46
Crackers, matzo, plain, 1 matzo	111	23	1	Tr	Tr	0	3	1
Crackers, melba toast, plain, 1 round	12	2	Tr	Tr	Tr	0	Tr	25
Crackers, rye, wafers, plain, 1 cracker	37	9	3	Tr	Tr	0	1	87
Crackers, saltines (oyster, soda, soup), 1 cup	195	32	1	5	1	0	4	586
Crackers, sandwich-type, with peanut butter filling, 1 sandwich	32	4	Tr	2	Tr	0	1	47
Crackers, wheat, 1 cracker	9	1	Tr	Tr	Tr	0	Tr	16

Food, portion	Calories	Total Carb (g)	Fiber (g)	Total Fat (g)	Sat Fat (g)	Chol (mg)	Protein (g)	Sodium (mg)
Croissants, butter, 1 croissant	231	26	1	12	7	38	5	424
Croutons, seasoned, 1 cup	186	25	2	7	2	3	4	495
Cupcake, creme-filled, chocolate with frosting, 1 cupcake	188	30	Tr	7	1	9	2	213
Danish pastry, cheese, 1 pastry	266	26	1	16	5	11	6	320
Doughnuts, cake-type, plain, chocolate-coated or frosted, 1 doughnut, 3" dia	204	21	1	13	3	26	2	184
Doughnuts, cake-type, plain, sugared or glazed, 1 doughnut, 3" dia	192	23	1	10	3	14	2	181
Doughnuts, yeast-leavened, glazed (includes honey buns), 1 doughnut, 3" dia	242	27	1	14	3	4	4	205
English muffins, plain, 1 muffin	134	26	2	1	Tr	0	4	264
English muffins, raisin-cinnamon (includes apple-cinnamon), 1 muffin	139	28	2	2	Tr	0	4	255
English muffins, wheat, 1 muffin	127	26	3	1	Tr	0	5	218
French toast, prepared from recipe, made with low-fat (2%) milk, 1 slice	149	16	na	7	2	75	5	311
Ice cream cones, wafer-type, 1 cone	17	3	Tr	Tr	Tr	0	Tr	6
Muffins, blueberry, 1 medium	313	54	3	7	2	34	6	505
Muffins, corn, 1 medium	345	58	4	9	2	29	7	589
Muffins, plain, prepared from recipe, with low-fat (2%) milk, 1 muffin	169	24	2	6	1	22	4	266
Pancakes, buttermilk, prepared from recipe, 1 pancake, 6" dia	175	22	na	7	1	45	5	402
Pancakes, plain, dry mix, complete, prepared, 1 pancake, 6" dia	149	28	1	2	Tr	9	4	484
Pie, apple, ⅛ of 9" dia pie	411	58	na	19	5	0	4	327
Pie, blueberry, ⅛ of 9" dia pie	290	44	1	13	2	0	2	406
Pie, chocolate creme, ¼ of 6" dia pie	301	33	2	19	5	5	3	135
Pie, pumpkin, ⅙ of 8" dia pie	229	30	3	10	2	22	4	307

FOOD, PORTION	CALORIES	TOTAL CARB (G)	FIBER (G)	TOTAL FAT (G)	SAT FAT (G)	CHOL (MG)	PROTEIN (G)	SODIUM (MG)
BAKED PRODUCTS *(CONT.)*								
Pita, white, 1 pita, 6½" dia	165	33	1	1	Tr	0	5	322
Popovers, dry mix, enriched, 1 oz	105	20	na	1	Tr	0	3	257
Rolls, dinner, French, 1 roll	105	19	1	2	Tr	0	3	231
Rolls, dinner, plain, 1 roll	84	14	1	2	Tr	Tr	2	146
Rolls, dinner, wheat, 1 roll	76	13	1	2	Tr	0	2	95
Rolls, dinner, whole-wheat, 1 hoagie roll	250	48	7	4	1	0	8	449
Rolls, hamburger or hotdog, plain, 1 roll	120	21	1	2	Tr	0	4	206
Rolls, hard (includes kaiser), 1 roll, 3½" dia	167	30	1	2	Tr	0	6	310
SHAKE 'N' BAKE original recipe, 1 serving	106	22	na	1	0	na	2	795
Strudel, apple, 1 piece	195	29	2	8	1	4	2	191
Taco shells, baked, 1 shell, approx 5" dia	62	8	1	3	Tr	0	1	49
Toaster pastries, fruit, 1 pastry	204	37	1	5	1	0	2	218
Tortillas, flour, 1 tortilla, approx 6" dia	104	18	1	2	1	0	3	153
Waffles, EGGO Golden Oat, 1 waffle	69	13	1	1	Tr	Tr	2	135
Waffles, EGGO Low-fat Homestyle, 1 waffle	83	15	Tr	1	Tr	9	2	155
Waffles, plain or buttermilk, ready-to-heat, 1 waffle	95	15	1	3	Tr	12	2	284
BEEF PRODUCTS								
Beef, ground, 95% lean/5% fat, pan-browned, 3 oz	164	0	0	6	3	76	25	72
Beef, ground, patties, frozen, broiled, medium, 3 oz	240	0	0	17	7	80	21	65
Breakfast strips, cured, cooked, 3 slices	153	Tr	0	12	5	40	11	766
Brisket, whole, braised, 3 oz	247	0	0	17	6	79	23	55
Chuck, top blade, broiled, 3 oz	173	0	0	9	3	51	22	58
Rib, eye, broiled, 3 oz	174	0	0	8	3	77	25	51
Rib, prime, broiled, 3 oz	250	0	0	18	8	70	21	60

Food, portion	Calories	Total Carb (g)	Fiber (g)	Total Fat (g)	Sat Fat (g)	Chol (mg)	Protein (g)	Sodium (mg)
Short loin, porterhouse steak, broiled, 3 oz	235	0	0	16	6	57	20	55
Short loin, T-bone steak, broiled, 3 oz	168	0	0	8	3	48	22	60
Tenderloin, broiled, 3 oz	175	0	0	8	0	78	25	50
Beverages								
Beer, light, 12 fl oz	99	5	0	0	0	0	1	11
Beer, regular, 12 fl oz	117	6	Tr	Tr	0	0	1	14
Carbonated beverage, low-calorie, other than cola or pepper, no caffeine, 12 fl oz	0	0	0	0	0	0	Tr	21
Chocolate syrup, 2 tbsp	109	25	1	Tr	Tr	0	1	28
Clam and tomato juice, canned, 5.5 oz	80	18	Tr	Tr	Tr	0	1	601
Club soda, 12 fl oz	0	0	0	0	0	0	0	75
Cocoa mix, powder, 1 serving	111	24	1	1	1	2	2	141
Coffee, brewed from grounds, 8 fl oz	9	0	0	2	0	0	Tr	2
Cola, 12 fl oz	155	40	0	0	0	0	Tr	15
Cranberry juice cocktail, bottled, 8 fl oz	144	36	Tr	Tr	Tr	0	0	5
Cream soda, 12 fl oz	189	49	0	0	0	0	0	45
Fruit punch juice drink, frozen concentrate, prepared with water, 8 fl oz	124	30	Tr	Tr	Tr	0	Tr	12
Ginger ale, 12 fl oz	124	32	0	0	0	0	0	26
Grape juice drink, 8 fl oz	125	32	0	0	0	0	Tr	3
KOOL-AID Tropical Punch, sweetened, powder, 1 serving	64	16	0	0	0	0	0	2
Lemonade, COUNTRY TIME, pink, sugar-free mix, 1 portion	5	2	na	Tr	0	na	Tr	Tr
Lemonade, frozen concentrate, white, prepared with water, 8 fl oz	131	34	Tr	Tr	Tr	0	Tr	7
NESTEA Ice Tea, Lemon Flavor, ready-to-drink, 8 fl oz	89	20	0	1	Tr	na	0	0
Orange juice drink, 8 fl oz	132	33	0	0	0	0	Tr	5

Food, portion	Calories	Total Carb (g)	Fiber (g)	Total Fat (g)	Sat Fat (g)	Chol (mg)	Protein (g)	Sodium (mg)
Beverages (cont.)								
Pepper-type cola, 12 fl oz	151	38	0	Tr	Tr	0	0	37
Pineapple and grapefruit juice drink, 8 fl oz	118	29	Tr	Tr	Tr	0	1	35
RICE DREAM, 8 fl oz	120	25	0	2	Tr	0	Tr	86
Root beer, 12 fl oz	152	39	0	0	0	0	0	48
Shake, chocolate, 8 fl oz	211	34	3	6	4	22	6	161
Shake, vanilla, 8 fl oz	184	30	Tr	5	3	18	6	136
Tea, brewed, 8 fl oz	2	1	0	0	Tr	0	0	7
Tea, instant, lemon flavor, prepared, 8 fl oz	5	1	0	0	0	0	Tr	24
Wine, table, red, 3.5 fl oz	74	2	0	0	0	0	Tr	5
Wine, table, white, 3.5 fl oz	70	1	0	0	0	0	Tr	5
Breakfast Cereals								
APPLE CINNAMON CHEERIOS, ¾ cup	118	25	1	2	Tr	0	2	120
BANANA NUT CRUNCH, 1 cup	249	44	4	6	1	0	5	253
BASIC 4, 1 cup	202	42	3	3	Tr	0	4	316
Bran flakes with raisins, 1 cup	187	46	8	1	Tr	0	5	360
CHEERIOS, 1 cup	111	22	3	2	Tr	0	3	273
CORN CHEX, 1 cup	112	26	1	Tr	Tr	0	2	288
CORN FLAKES, 1 cup	101	24	1	Tr	Tr	0	2	203
CORN POPS, 1 cup	118	28	Tr	Tr	Tr	0	1	120
CREAM OF RICE, cooked with water, 1 tbsp	8	2	Tr	Tr	Tr	0	Tr	Tr
CREAM OF WHEAT, instant, prepared with water, 1 cup	149	32	1	1	Tr	0	4	10
CRISPIX, 1 cup	109	25	Tr	Tr	Tr	0	2	210
FIBER ONE, ½ cup	59	24	14	1	Tr	0	2	129
FROSTED FLAKES, ¾ cup	114	28	1	Tr	Tr	0	1	148
FROSTED WHEATIES, ¾ cup	112	27	1	Tr	Tr	0	2	204
GOLDEN GRAHAMS, ¾ cup	112	25	1	1	Tr	0	2	269

Food, portion	Calories	Total Carb (g)	Fiber (g)	Total Fat (g)	Sat Fat (g)	Chol (mg)	Protein (g)	Sodium (mg)
HONEY BUNCHES OF OATS, ¾ cup	118	25	1	2	Tr	0	2	193
HONEY NUT CHEERIOS, 1 cup	112	24	2	1	Tr	0	3	269
Multi-Bran CHEX, 1 cup	166	41	6	1	Tr	0	3	322
POST 100% BRAN, ⅓ cup	83	23	8	1	Tr	0	4	121
POST GRAPE-NUTS, ½ cup	208	47	5	1	Tr	0	6	354
PRODUCT 19, 1 cup	100	25	1	Tr	Tr	0	2	207
QUAKER Instant Oatmeal, apples and cinnamon, 1 packet, prepared	130	26	3	1	Tr	0	3	165
RAISIN BRAN, 1 cup	195	47	7	2	Tr	0	5	362
RAISIN NUT BRAN, 1 cup	209	41	5	4	1	0	5	250
RICE KRISPIES, 1¼ cups	119	29	Tr	Tr	Tr	0	2	319
SPECIAL K, 1 cup	117	22	1	Tr	Tr	0	7	224
TOTAL Corn Flakes, 1⅓ cups	112	26	1	Tr	Tr	0	2	209
TRIX, 1 cup	117	27	1	1	Tr	0	1	194
WHEATIES, 1 cup	107	24	3	1	Tr	0	3	218
Whole-Grain TOTAL, ¾ cup	97	23	2	1	Tr	0	2	192
CEREAL GRAINS AND PASTA								
Barley, 1 cup	651	135	32	4	1	0	23	22
Corn flour, whole-grain, yellow, 1 cup	422	90	16	5	1	0	8	6
Cornmeal, whole-grain, yellow, 1 cup	442	94	9	4	1	0	10	43
Couscous, cooked, 1 cup	176	36	2	Tr	Tr	0	6	8
Macaroni, cooked, 1 cup small shells	162	33	1	1	Tr	0	5	1
Noodles, Chinese, chow mein, 1 cup	237	26	2	14	2	0	4	198
Noodles, egg, cooked, enriched, 1 cup	213	40	2	2	Tr	53	8	11
Noodles, somen, cooked, 1 cup	231	48	na	Tr	Tr	0	7	283
Oat bran, cooked, 1 cup	88	25	6	2	Tr	0	7	2
Pasta, corn, cooked, 1 cup	176	39	7	1	Tr	0	4	na

Food, portion	Calories	Total Carb (g)	Fiber (g)	Total Fat (g)	Sat Fat (g)	Chol (mg)	Protein (g)	Sodium (mg)
CEREAL GRAINS AND PASTAS (CONT.)								
Pasta, fresh-refrigerated, cooked, 2 oz	75	14	na	1	Tr	19	3	3
Rice, brown, long-grain, cooked, 1 cup	216	45	4	2	Tr	0	5	10
Rice flour, white, 1 cup	578	127	4	2	1	0	9	na
Rice noodles, cooked, 1 cup	192	44	2	Tr	Tr	0	2	33
Rice, white, cooked, 1 cup	169	37	2	Tr	Tr	0	4	9
Rice, white, long-grain, cooked, 1 cup	205	45	1	Tr	Tr	0	4	2
Rye flour, medium, 1 cup	361	79	15	2	Tr	0	10	3
Spaghetti, cooked, enriched, 1 cup	197	40	2	1	Tr	0	7	1
Wheat flour, white, enriched, 1 cup	455	95	3	1	Tr	0	13	3
Wheat flour, whole-grain, 1 cup	407	87	15	2	Tr	0	16	6
Wild rice, cooked, 1 cup	166	35	3	1	Tr	0	7	5
DAIRY AND EGG PRODUCTS								
Butter, salted, 1 tbsp	102	Tr	0	12	6	31	Tr	82
Butter, without salt, 1 tbsp	102	Tr	0	12	7	31	Tr	2
Cheese, American, 1 oz	94	2	0	7	4	18	6	274
Cheese, blue, 1 cup, crumbled	477	3	0	39	25	101	29	1883
Cheese, brick, 1 oz	105	1	0	8	5	27	7	159
Cheese, cheddar, 1 slice	113	Tr	0	9	6	29	7	174
Cheese, cream, 1 tbsp	51	Tr	0	5	3	16	1	43
Cheese, cream, low-fat, 1 tbsp	35	1	0	3	2	8	2	44
Cheese, feta, 1 cup, crumbled	396	6	0	32	22	134	21	1674
Cheese, gouda, 1 oz	101	1	0	8	5	32	7	232
Cheese, Mexican, queso anejo, 1 oz	106	1	0	8	5	30	6	321
Cheese, mozzarella, part-skim milk, 1 oz	72	1	0	5	3	18	7	175
Cheese, parmesan, grated, 1 cup	431	4	0	29	17	88	38	1529
Cheese, provolone, 1 slice	98	1	0	7	5	19	7	245

Food, portion	Calories	Total Carb (g)	Fiber (g)	Total Fat (g)	Sat Fat (g)	Chol (mg)	Protein (g)	Sodium (mg)
Cheese, Swiss, 1 slice	106	2	0	8	5	26	8	54
Cheese, Swiss, low-fat, 1 slice	50	1	0	1	1	10	8	73
CHEEZ WHIZ cheese sauce, 2 tbsp	91	3	Tr	7	4	25	4	541
Cottage cheese, low-fat, 2% milkfat, 1 cup	203	8	0	4	3	18	31	918
Cream, half-and-half, 1 fl oz	39	1	0	3	2	11	1	12
Cream, light (coffee or table cream), 1 fl oz	59	1	0	6	4	20	1	12
Cream, sour, cultured, 1 tbsp	26	1	0	3	2	5	Tr	6
Cream, sour, reduced-fat, 1 tbsp	20	1	0	2	1	6	Tr	6
Dessert topping, pressurized, 1 tbsp	11	1	0	1	1	0	Tr	2
Egg, white only, raw, fresh, 1 large	17	Tr	0	Tr	0	0	4	55
Egg, whole, hard-boiled, 1 large	78	1	0	5	2	212	6	62
Egg, whole, omelet, 1 large	93	Tr	0	7	2	217	6	98
Egg, whole, scrambled, 1 large	101	1	0	7	2	215	7	171
Egg, yolk only, raw, fresh, 1 large	55	1	0	5	2	210	3	8
Eggnog, 1 cup	343	34	0	19	11	150	10	137
Egg substitute, liquid, 1 cup	211	2	0	8	2	3	30	444
KRAFT FREE Singles, American, nonfat, 1 slice	31	2	Tr	Tr	Tr	3	5	273
Milk, 2% milkfat, added vitamin A, 1 cup	122	11	0	5	2	20	8	115
Milk, whole, 3.25% milkfat, 1 cup	146	11	0	8	5	24	8	105
Milk, imitation, nonsoy, 1 cup	112	13	0	5	1	0	4	134
Milk, nonfat, added vitamin A, 1 cup	83	12	0	Tr	Tr	5	8	108
Yogurt, fruit variety, nonfat, 8 oz	213	43	0	Tr	Tr	5	10	132
Yogurt, plain, low-fat, 8 oz	143	16	0	4	2	14	12	159
Yogurt, vanilla, low-fat, 8 oz	193	31	0	3	2	11	11	150
Fast Foods								
Biscuit, with egg and ham, 1 biscuit	442	30	1	27	6	300	20	1382
Biscuit with egg and sausage, 1 biscuit	581	41	1	39	15	302	19	1141

Food, portion	Calories	Total Carb (g)	Fiber (g)	Total Fat (g)	Sat Fat (g)	Chol (mg)	Protein (g)	Sodium (mg)
Fast Foods *(cont.)*								
Biscuit, with sausage, 1 biscuit	485	40	1	32	14	35	12	1071
Burrito, bean and cheese, 2 pieces	378	55	na	12	7	28	15	1166
Burrito, bean, cheese, and beef, 2 pieces	331	40	na	13	7	124	15	991
Cheeseburger, large, double patty, with condiments and vegetables, 1 sandwich	704	40	na	44	18	142	38	1148
Cheeseburger, large, single patty, with condiments and vegetables, 1 sandwich	563	38	na	33	15	88	28	1108
Chicken, breaded and fried, boneless pieces, plain, 6 pieces	319	15	0	21	5	61	18	513
Chicken, breaded and fried, boneless pieces, with bbq sauce, 6 pieces	330	25	na	18	6	61	17	829
Chicken, breaded and fried, light meat (breast or wing), 2 pieces	494	20	na	30	8	148	36	975
Chicken fillet sandwich, plain, 1 sandwich	515	39	na	29	9	60	24	957
Chili con carne, 1 cup	256	22	na	8	3	134	25	1007
Coleslaw, ¾ cup	147	13	na	11	2	5	1	267
Corn on the cob with butter, 1 ear	155	32	na	3	2	6	4	29
Croissant, with egg, cheese, and sausage, 1 croissant	523	25	na	38	18	216	20	1115
Egg and cheese sandwich, 1 sandwich	340	26	na	19	7	291	16	804
Enchilada, cheese and beef, 1 enchilada	323	30	na	18	9	40	12	1319
English muffin, with egg, cheese, and sausage, 1 muffin	487	31	na	31	12	274	22	1135
Fish fillet, battered or breaded, fried, 1 fillet	211	15	Tr	11	3	31	13	484
Fish sandwich, with tartar sauce, 1 sandwich	431	41	na	23	5	55	17	615
French toast with butter, 2 slices	356	36	na	19	8	116	10	513
Ham and cheese sandwich, 1 sandwich	352	33	na	15	6	58	21	771
Hamburger, large, double patty, with condiments and vegetables, 1 sandwich	540	40	na	27	11	122	34	791

Food, portion	Calories	Total Carb (g)	Fiber (g)	Total Fat (g)	Sat Fat (g)	Chol (mg)	Protein (g)	Sodium (mg)
Hamburger, large, single patty, with condiments, 1 sandwich	427	37	2	21	8	71	23	731
Hot dog, plain, 1 sandwich	242	18	na	15	5	44	10	670
Nachos, with cheese, 6–8 nachos	346	36	na	19	8	18	9	816
Pizza with cheese, meat, and vegetables, 1 slice	184	21	na	5	2	21	13	382
Pizza with pepperoni, 1 slice	181	20	na	7	2	14	10	267
Potato, baked and topped with cheese sauce and broccoli, 1 piece	403	47	na	21	9	20	14	485
Potato, french fried in vegetable oil, 1 medium	458	53	5	25	5	0	6	265
Potato salad, ⅓ cup	108	13	na	6	1	57	1	312
Roast beef sandwich, plain, 1 sandwich	346	33	na	14	4	51	22	792
Salad, vegetable, tossed, without dressing, with chicken, 1½ cups	105	4	na	2	1	72	17	209
Salad, vegetable, tossed, without dressing, with pasta and seafood, 1½ cups	379	32	na	21	3	50	16	1572
Shrimp, breaded and fried, 6–8 shrimp	454	40	na	25	5	200	19	1446
Steak sandwich, 1 sandwich	459	52	na	14	4	73	30	798
Submarine sandwich, with cold cuts, 1 sub	456	51	na	19	7	36	22	1651
Sundae, hot fudge, 1 sundae	284	48	0	9	5	21	6	182
Taco, 1 large	568	41	na	32	17	87	32	1233
Taco salad, 1½ cups	279	24	na	15	7	44	13	762
Fats and Oils								
Bacon grease, 1 tsp	39	0	0	4	2	4	0	6
Fish oil, sardine, 1 tbsp	123	0	0	14	4	97	0	na
Lard, 1 tbsp	115	0	0	13	5	12	0	na
Margarine, 80% fat, stick, 1 tbsp	99	Tr	0	11	2	0	Tr	92
Margarine spread, fat-free, tub, 1 tbsp	6	1	0	Tr	Tr	0	Tr	85

Food, portion	Calories	Total Carb (g)	Fiber (g)	Total Fat (g)	Sat Fat (g)	Chol (mg)	Protein (g)	Sodium (mg)
Fats and Oils (cont.)								
Margarine, spread, soybean, 1 tbsp	87	Tr	na	10	2	0	Tr	98
Margarine-butter blend, 60% corn oil margarine and 40% butter, 1 tbsp	102	Tr	0	11	4	12	Tr	127
Mayonnaise dressing, no cholesterol, 1 tbsp	103	Tr	0	12	2	0	0	73
Mayonnaise, made with tofu, 1 tbsp	48	1	Tr	5	Tr	0	1	116
MIRACLE WHIP FREE, nonfat, 1 tbsp	13	2	Tr	Tr	Tr	1	Tr	126
Oil, canola, 1 tbsp	124	0	0	14	1	0	0	na
Oil, corn, 1 tbsp	120	0	0	14	2	0	0	na
Oil, olive, 1 tbsp	119	0	0	14	2	0	0	Tr
Oil, soybean, 1 tbsp	120	0	0	14	2	0	0	na
Salad dressing, Caesar, 1 tbsp	78	Tr	Tr	8	1	Tr	Tr	158
Salad dressing, French, 1 tbsp	73	2	0	7	1	0	Tr	134
Salad dressing, Italian, 1 tbsp	43	2	0	4	1	0	Tr	243
Salad dressing, peppercorn, 1 tbsp	76	Tr	0	8	1	7	Tr	143
Salad dressing, thousand island, 1 tbsp	59	2	Tr	6	1	4	Tr	138
Salad dressing, vinegar and oil, 1 tbsp	72	Tr	0	8	1	0	0	Tr
Finfish and Shellfish Products								
Anchovy, European, canned in oil, drained, 1 anchovy	8	0	0	Tr	Tr	3	1	147
Catfish, breaded and fried, 3 oz	195	7	1	11	3	69	15	238
Clam, breaded and fried, 20 small	380	19	na	21	5	115	27	684
Clam, canned, drained, 3 oz	126	4	0	2	Tr	57	22	95
Cod, Atlantic, cooked, dry heat, 3 oz	89	0	0	1	Tr	47	19	66
Crab, Alaska king, cooked, moist heat, 1 leg	130	0	0	2	Tr	71	26	1436
Crab, queen, cooked, 3 oz	98	0	0	1	Tr	60	20	587
Fish sticks, frozen, preheated, 1 stick	76	7	Tr	3	1	31	4	163
Flounder and sole, cooked, dry heat, 3 oz	99	0	0	1	Tr	58	21	89

Food, portion	Calories	Total Carb (g)	Fiber (g)	Total Fat (g)	Sat Fat (g)	Chol (mg)	Protein (g)	Sodium (mg)
Halibut, cooked, dry heat, 3 oz	119	0	0	2	Tr	35	23	59
Herring, Pacific, cooked, dry heat, 3 oz	213	0	0	15	4	84	18	81
Lobster, northern, cooked, 3 oz	83	1	0	1	Tr	61	17	323
Mackerel, king, cooked, 3 oz	114	0	0	2	Tr	58	22	173
Ocean perch, cooked, dry heat, 3 oz	103	0	0	2	Tr	46	20	82
Oyster, wild, cooked, moist heat, 3 oz	116	7	0	4	1	89	12	359
Pike, northern, cooked, dry heat, 3 oz	96	0	0	1	Tr	43	21	42
Roe, mixed, cooked, dry heat, 3 oz	173	2	0	7	2	407	24	99
Roughy, orange, cooked, dry heat, 3 oz	76	0	0	1	Tr	22	16	69
Salmon, Atlantic, farmed, cooked, 3 oz	175	0	0	10	2	54	19	52
Sardine, Atlantic, canned in oil, drained solids with bone, 2 sardines	50	0	0	3	Tr	34	6	121
Scallop, breaded and fried, 2 large	67	3	na	3	1	19	6	144
Shrimp, mixed, breaded and fried, 3 oz	206	10	Tr	10	2	150	18	292
Shrimp, mixed, cooked, moist heat, 3 oz	84	0	0	1	Tr	166	18	190
Snapper, mixed, cooked, dry heat, 3 oz	109	0	0	1	Tr	40	22	48
Surimi, 3 oz	84	6	0	1	Tr	26	13	122
Swordfish, cooked, dry heat, 3 oz	132	0	0	4	1	43	22	98
Trout, rainbow, wild, cooked, dry heat, 3 oz	128	0	0	5	1	59	19	48
Tuna, light, canned in water, drained, 1 can	191	0	0	1	Tr	50	42	558
Tuna salad, 3 oz	159	8	0	8	1	11	14	342
Fruits and Fruit Juices								
Apple juice, canned or bottled, unsweetened, 1 cup	117	29	Tr	Tr	Tr	0	Tr	7
Apples, canned, sweetened, sliced, 1 cup	137	34	3	1	Tr	0	Tr	6
Apples, with skin, 1 apple, 2¾" dia	72	19	3	Tr	Tr	0	Tr	1
Applesauce, canned, sweetened, 1 cup	194	51	3	Tr	Tr	0	Tr	8
Bananas, 1 banana, 7" to 7⅞" long	105	27	3	Tr	Tr	0	1	1

FRUITS AND FRUIT JUICES (CONT.)

Food, portion	Calories	Total Carb (g)	Fiber (g)	Total Fat (g)	Sat Fat (g)	Chol (mg)	Protein (g)	Sodium (mg)
Blackberries, 1 cup	62	14	8	1	Tr	0	2	1
Blueberries, 1 cup	83	21	3	Tr	Tr	0	1	1
Cantaloupe, 1/8 of melon	35	8	1	Tr	Tr	0	1	16
Casaba, 1 cup, cubes	48	11	2	Tr	Tr	0	2	15
Cherries, sweet, 1 cup, with pits	74	19	2	Tr	Tr	0	1	na
Cranberry juice, unsweetened, 1 cup	116	31	Tr	Tr	Tr	0	1	5
Cranberry sauce, canned, sweetened, 1 cup	418	108	3	Tr	Tr	0	1	80
Dates, deglet noor, 1 date	23	6	1	Tr	Tr	0	Tr	Tr
Figs, 1 fig, 2¼" dia	37	10	1	Tr	Tr	0	Tr	1
Fruit cocktail (peach, pineapple, pear, grape, cherry), juice pack, 1 cup	109	28	2	Tr	Tr	0	1	9
Grapefruit juice, white, canned, sweetened, 1 cup	115	28	Tr	Tr	Tr	0	1	5
Grapefruit, pink and red, ½ fruit, 3¾" dia	37	9	1	Tr	Tr	0	1	na
Grapes, red or green, 1 grape, seedless	3	1	Tr	Tr	Tr	0	Tr	Tr
Honeydew, 1/8 of a melon	45	11	1	Tr	Tr	0	1	23
Kiwi fruit, fresh, 1 fruit without skin	56	13	3	Tr	Tr	0	1	3
Kumquats, 1 fruit	13	3	1	Tr	Tr	0	Tr	2
Lemons, without peel, 1 fruit, 2⅜" dia	24	8	2	Tr	Tr	0	1	2
Limes, 1 fruit, 2" dia	15	6	2	Tr	Tr	0	Tr	1
Mangos, 1 fruit	135	35	4	1	Tr	0	1	4
Nectarines, 1 fruit, 2½" dia	60	14	2	Tr	Tr	0	1	na
Olives, ripe, canned, 1 large olive	5	Tr	Tr	Tr	Tr	0	Tr	38
Orange juice, canned, unsweetened, 1 cup	105	25	Tr	Tr	Tr	0	1	5
Orange-grapefruit juice, canned, unsweetened, 1 cup	106	25	Tr	Tr	Tr	0	1	7
Oranges, 1 fruit, 2⅝" dia	62	15	3	Tr	Tr	0	1	na

FOOD, PORTION	CALORIES	TOTAL CARB (G)	FIBER (G)	TOTAL FAT (G)	SAT FAT (G)	CHOL (MG)	PROTEIN (G)	SODIUM (MG)
Papayas, 1 fruit, 5⅛" long×3" dia	119	30	5	Tr	Tr	0	2	9
Peaches, canned, juice pack, 1 cup, halves	109	29	3	Tr	Tr	0	2	10
Peaches, 1 fruit, 2½" dia	38	9	1	Tr	Tr	0	1	na
Pears, 1 fruit, approx 2½ per lb	96	26	5	Tr	Tr	0	1	2
Pineapple, canned, juice pack, drained, 1 cup, chunks	109	28	2	Tr	Tr	0	1	2
Pineapple juice, canned, unsweetened, 1 cup	140	34	1	Tr	Tr	0	1	3
Pineapple, 1 slice, 3½" dia×½" thick	27	7	1	Tr	Tr	0	Tr	1
Plums, 1 fruit, 2⅛" dia	30	8	1	Tr	Tr	0	Tr	na
Prune juice, canned, 1 cup	182	45	3	Tr	Tr	0	2	10
Prunes, uncooked, 1 cup, pitted	408	109	12	1	Tr	0	4	3
Raisins, seedless, ½ oz box	42	11	1	Tr	Tr	0	Tr	2
Raspberries, 1 cup	64	15	8	1	Tr	0	1	1
Rhubarb, 1 cup, diced	26	6	2	Tr	Tr	0	1	5
Strawberries, 1 cup, whole	46	11	3	Tr	Tr	0	1	1
Tangerines, 1 fruit, 2⅜" dia	37	9	2	Tr	Tr	0	1	1
Watermelon, approx 1/16 of melon	86	22	1	Tr	Tr	0	2	3
LAMB AND VEAL PRODUCTS								
Lamb, ground, broiled, 3 oz	241	0	0	17	7	82	21	69
Lamb, leg, (shank and sirloin), roasted, 3 oz	162	0	na	7	3	76	23	61
Veal, ground, broiled, 3 oz	146	0	0	6	3	88	21	71
Veal, loin, roasted, 3 oz	184	0	0	10	4	88	21	79
Veal, rib, braised, 3 oz	185	0	0	7	2	122	29	84
Veal, sirloin, braised, 3 oz	214	0	0	11	4	92	27	67
LEGUMES AND LEGUME PRODUCTS								
Bacon, meatless, 1 strip	16	Tr	Tr	1	Tr	0	1	73
Bacon bits, meatless, 1 tbsp	33	2	1	2	Tr	0	2	124

LEGUMES AND LEGUME PRODUCTS (CONT.)

FOOD, PORTION	CALORIES	TOTAL CARB (G)	FIBER (G)	TOTAL FAT (G)	SAT FAT (G)	CHOL (MG)	PROTEIN (G)	SODIUM (MG)
Beans, baked, canned, 1 cup	236	52	13	1	Tr	0	12	1008
Beans, baked, canned, with beef, 1 cup	322	45	na	9	4	59	17	1264
Beans, baked, canned, with franks, 1 cup	368	40	18	17	6	16	17	1114
Beans, black, boiled, 1 cup	227	41	15	1	Tr	0	15	2
Beans, kidney, red, boiled, 1 cup	225	40	13	1	Tr	0	15	4
Beans, navy, boiled, 1 cup	258	48	12	1	Tr	0	16	2
Chili with beans, canned, 1 cup	287	30	11	14	6	44	15	1336
Cowpeas (blackeyes, crowder, southern), boiled, 1 cup	200	36	11	1	Tr	0	13	7
Falafel, home-prepared, 1 patty, 2¼" dia	57	5	na	3	Tr	0	2	50
GREEN GIANT, HARVEST BURGER, 1 patty	138	7	6	4	1	0	18	411
Hummus, commercial, 1 cup	415	36	15	24	4	0	20	948
Lentils, boiled, 1 cup	230	40	16	1	Tr	0	18	4
Lima beans, boiled, 1 cup	216	39	13	1	Tr	0	15	4
MORI-NU, Tofu, silken, soft, 1 slice	46	2	Tr	2	Tr	0	4	4
Peanut butter, chunk style, with salt, 2 tbsp	188	7	2	16	3	0	8	150
Peanut butter, smooth style, with salt, 2 tbsp	192	6	2	17	3	0	8	160
Peanuts, dry-roasted, without salt, 1 cup	854	31	12	73	10	0	35	9
Peanuts, raw, 1 cup	828	24	12	72	10	0	38	26
Peas, split, boiled, 1 cup	231	41	16	1	Tr	0	16	4
Refried beans, canned, 1 cup	237	39	13	3	1	20	14	753
Soy milk, 1 cup	120	11	3	5	1	0	9	29
Soy sauce, soy (tamari), 1 tbsp	11	1	Tr	Tr	Tr	0	2	1005
Soybeans, boiled, with salt, 1 cup	298	17	10	15	2	0	29	408
Soyburger, 1 patty	125	9	3	4	1	0	13	385
Tofu, fried, 1 piece	35	1	1	3	Tr	0	2	2

FOOD, PORTION	CALORIES	TOTAL CARB (G)	FIBER (G)	TOTAL FAT (G)	SAT FAT (G)	CHOL (MG)	PROTEIN (G)	SODIUM (MG)
Vegetarian fillets, 1 fillet	247	8	5	15	2	0	20	417
Vegetarian stew, 1 cup	304	17	3	7	1	0	42	988
MEALS, ENTRÉES, AND SIDE DISHES								
BANQUET Chicken Pot Pie, frozen, 1 serving	382	36	1	22	9	40	10	948
BANQUET Turkey & Gravy with Dressing Meal, frozen meal, 1 serving	280	34	3	10	3	52	14	1061
Beef stew, canned, 1 serving	218	16	3	12	5	37	11	947
Breakfast Burrito, Ham & Cheese, frozen entrée, 1 serving	212	28	1	7	2	192	10	405
CHEF BOYARDEE Spaghetti & Meatballs in Tomato Sauce, 1 serving	250	34	2	9	4	22	9	941
CHUN KING Sweet & Sour Vegetables & Sauce with Chicken, canned, 1 serving	165	32	na	2	0	23	6	564
Cinnamon Swirl French Toast with Sausage, 1 serving	415	38	2	23	7	98	13	502
DINTY MOORE Beef Stew, 1 serving	222	16	3	13	6	38	11	984
GREEN GIANT, Broccoli in Cheese Flavored Sauce, frozen, 1 serving	75	10	na	3	1	0	3	538
HAMBURGER HELPER, Cheeseburger Macaroni, dry mix, 1 serving	178	29	na	5	1	4	5	914
HEALTHY CHOICE Chicken Teriyaki with Rice Medley, frozen meal, 1 serving	268	37	3	6	3	44	17	602
HORMEL Chili with Beans, 1 cup	240	34	8	4	2	25	17	1163
HOT POCKETS Ham 'N Cheese, frozen, 1 serving	340	38	na	14	6	50	15	666
KRAFT Macaroni and Cheese Dinner Original Flavor, unprepared, 1 serving	259	48	1	3	1	10	11	561
LEAN CUISINE Rice and Chicken Stir-Fry with Vegetables, frozen entrée, 1 serving	270	40	6	7	1	26	12	632
LIPTON, Alfredo Egg Noodles in a Creamy Sauce, dry mix, 1 serving	259	39	na	7	3	69	10	1097

Food, portion	Calories	Total Carb (g)	Fiber (g)	Total Fat (g)	Sat Fat (g)	Chol (mg)	Protein (g)	Sodium (mg)
Meals, Entrées, and Side Dishes (cont.)								
MARIE CALLENDER'S Escalloped Noodles & Chicken, frozen entrée, 1 cup	397	38	na	21	7	na	13	1007
OLD EL PASO Chili with Beans, 1 serving	249	22	10	10	2	36	18	588
STOUFFER'S Creamed Spinach, frozen, 1 serving	169	9	2	13	4	16	4	335
THE BUDGET GOURMET Italian Sausage Lasagna, frozen entrée, 1 serving	456	40	3	24	8	48	21	903
Tortellini, pasta with cheese filling, ¾ cup	249	38	2	6	3	34	11	279
TYSON Beef Stir Fry Kit, frozen, 1 serving	433	71	na	5	0	na	26	1584
TYSON Chicken Fajita Kit, frozen, 1 serving	129	17	na	3	1	13	8	350
Nut and Seed Products								
Almonds, 1 cup, whole	827	28	17	72	6	0	30	1
Coconut meat, dried, sweetened, flaked, 1 cup	351	35	3	24	21	0	2	189
Hazelnuts or filberts, 1 cup, whole	848	23	13	82	6	0	20	na
Macadamia nuts, dry roasted, 1 cup, whole	962	18	11	102	16	0	10	5
Mixed nuts, peanuts, dry roasted, salted, 1 cup	814	35	12	70	9	0	24	917
Pecans, 1 cup, halves	684	14	10	71	6	0	9	na
Pistachio nuts, dry roasted, salted, 1 cup	699	33	13	57	7	0	26	498
Sunflower seed kernels, dried, 1 cup	821	27	15	71	7	0	33	4
Walnuts, English, 1 cup, pieces	785	16	8	78	7	0	18	2
Pork Products								
Bacon, cured, pan-fried, 1 slice cooked	42	Tr	0	3	1	9	3	192
Canadian bacon, cured, grilled, 2 slices	87	1	0	4	1	27	11	727
Ham, boneless, approx 11% fat, roasted, 3 oz	151	0	0	8	3	50	19	1275
Ham, cured, boneless, extra lean, roasted, 3 oz	140	Tr	0	7	2	48	19	1177
Ham, leg, shank half, roasted, 3 oz	246	0	0	17	6	78	22	50
Pork, fresh, ground, cooked, 3 oz	252	0	0	18	7	80	22	62

Food, portion	Calories	Total Carb (g)	Fiber (g)	Total Fat (g)	Sat Fat (g)	Chol (mg)	Protein (g)	Sodium (mg)
Pork, sirloin (chops), boneless, braised, 3 oz	149	0	0	6	2	69	23	39
Pork, tenderloin, roasted, 3 oz	147	0	0	5	2	67	24	47
Poultry Products								
Chicken, breast, meat and skin, batter-fried, ½ breast, bone removed	364	13	Tr	18	5	119	35	385
Chicken, dark meat and skin, roasted, ½ chicken, bone removed	423	0	0	26	7	152	43	145
Chicken, drumstick, meat and skin, batter-fried, 1 drumstick, bone removed	193	6	Tr	11	3	62	16	194
Chicken, leg, meat and skin, roasted, 1 leg, bone removed	264	0	0	15	4	105	30	99
Chicken, light meat and skin, batter-fried, ½ chicken, bone removed	521	18	na	29	8	158	44	540
Chicken, thigh, meat and skin, roasted, 1 thigh, bone removed	153	0	0	10	3	58	16	52
Chicken, wing, meat and skin, batter-fried, 1 wing, bone removed	159	5	Tr	11	3	39	10	157
Cornish game hens, meat and skin, roasted, 1 bird	668	0	0	47	13	337	57	164
Ground turkey, cooked, 4 oz raw patty	193	0	0	11	3	84	22	88
Turkey, breast, meat and skin, roasted, ½ breast, bone removed	1633	0	0	64	18	639	248	544
Turkey, leg, meat and skin, roasted, 1 leg	148	0	0	7	2	60	20	55
Turkey, wing, meat and skin, roasted, 1 wing, bone removed	426	0	0	23	6	151	51	113
Sausages and Luncheon Meats								
Beef, cured, pastrami, 1 oz	98	1	0	8	3	26	5	344
Beef, sausage, smoked, 1 sausage	134	1	0	12	5	29	6	486
Bologna, beef, 1 serving	87	1	0	8	3	16	3	302
Bologna, turkey, 1 serving	59	1	Tr	4	1	21	3	351

Food, portion	Calories	Total Carb (g)	Fiber (g)	Total Fat (g)	Sat Fat (g)	Chol (mg)	Protein (g)	Sodium (mg)
Sausages and Luncheon Meats (cont.)								
Chicken breast, oven-roasted, fat-free, sliced, 1 serving	33	1	0	Tr	Tr	15	7	457
Frankfurter, beef, 5" long×¾" dia	149	2	0	13	5	24	5	513
Ham, sliced, approx 11% fat, 1 slice	46	1	Tr	2	1	16	5	365
Pastrami, beef, 98% fat-free, 1 serving	54	1	0	1	0	27	11	576
Pepperoni, pork, beef, 1 oz	130	1	Tr	11	5	33	6	501
Salami, cooked, beef, 1 slice	67	Tr	0	6	3	18	3	296
Sausage, Italian, pork, cooked, 1 link	268	1	0	21	8	65	17	765
Sausage, Polish, pork and beef, smoked, 1 serving	229	2	0	20	7	54	9	644
SPAM, pork with ham, minced, 1 serving	174	2	0	15	6	39	7	767
Turkey sausage, reduced-fat, brown-and-serve, 1 cup	256	14	Tr	13	4	74	22	790
Snacks								
Banana chips, 3 oz	441	50	7	29	25	0	2	5
Beef jerky, 1 piece	82	2	Tr	5	2	10	7	443
Cheese puffs and twists, low-fat, 1 oz	122	21	3	3	1	Tr	2	364
CHEX mix, 1 oz	120	18	2	5	2	0	3	288
Granola bars, soft, uncoated, chocolate chip, 1 bar	118	19	1	5	3	Tr	2	76
Granola bars, soft, uncoated, plain, 1 bar	124	19	1	5	2	Tr	2	78
Popcorn, air-popped, 1 cup	31	6	1	Tr	Tr	0	1	Tr
Popcorn, caramel-coated, with peanuts, 1 oz	113	23	1	2	Tr	0	2	84
Potato chips, barbecue-flavor, 1 bag, 7 oz	972	105	9	64	16	0	15	1485
Potato chips, plain, salted, 1 bag, 8 oz	1217	120	10	79	25	0	16	1348
Pretzels, hard, plain, unsalted, 10 twists	229	48	2	2	Tr	0	5	173
Pretzels, soft, 1 medium	389	80	2	4	1	3	9	1615
Puffs, corn-based, cheese-flavor, 8 oz	1258	122	2	78	15	9	17	2384

FOOD, PORTION	CALORIES	TOTAL CARB (G)	FIBER (G)	TOTAL FAT (G)	SAT FAT (G)	CHOL (MG)	PROTEIN (G)	SODIUM (MG)
Rice cake, cracker, 1 cubic inch	16	3	Tr	Tr	Tr	0	Tr	3
Sesame sticks, wheat-based, salted, 1 oz	153	13	1	10	2	0	3	422
Tortilla chips, plain, 1 oz	142	18	2	7	1	0	2	150
Trail mix, regular, 1 cup	693	67	na	44	8	0	21	344
Trail mix, with chocolate chips, salted nuts, and seeds, 1 cup	707	66	na	47	9	6	21	177
SOUPS, SAUCES, AND GRAVIES								
Barbecue sauce, 1 cup (8 fl oz)	188	32	3	5	1	0	5	2038
CHEF-MATE Basic Cheddar Cheese Sauce, 1 serving	82	8	0	5	2	6	2	471
Gravy, beef, canned, 1 cup	123	11	1	5	3	7	9	1305
Gravy, turkey, canned, 1 cup	121	12	1	5	1	5	6	1373
LJ MINOR Stir Fry Sauce, 1 serving	16	2	0	1	Tr	0	Tr	233
LJ MINOR Sweet N' Sour Sauce, 1 serving	40	8	Tr	1	Tr	0	Tr	116
LJ MINOR Teriyaki Sauce, 1 serving	21	4	0	1	Tr	0	Tr	159
Sauce, pasta, spaghetti/marinara, ready-to-serve, 1 cup	143	21	4	5	1	0	4	1030
Soup, black bean, canned, prepared with equal volume water, 1 cup	116	20	4	2	Tr	0	6	1198
Soup, chicken noodle, canned, prepared with equal volume water, 1 cup	75	9	1	2	1	7	4	1106
Soup, chicken vegetable, canned, prepared with equal volume water, 1 cup	75	9	1	3	1	10	4	945
Soup, cream of chicken, prepared with equal volume milk, 1 cup	191	15	Tr	11	5	27	7	1047
Soup, cream of potato, canned, prepared with equal volume milk, 1 cup	149	17	Tr	6	4	22	6	1061
Soup, lentil with ham, canned, 1 cup	139	20	na	3	1	7	9	1319
Soup, onion, canned, condensed, 1 cup	113	16	2	3	1	0	8	2116

Food, portion	Calories	Total Carb (g)	Fiber (g)	Total Fat (g)	Sat Fat (g)	Chol (mg)	Protein (g)	Sodium (mg)
Soups, Sauces, and Gravies *(cont.)*								
Soup, pea, green, canned, prepared with equal volume milk, 1 cup	239	32	3	7	4	18	13	970
Soup, tomato, canned, prepared with equal volume water, 1 cup	85	17	Tr	2	Tr	0	2	695
Soup, vegetarian vegetable, canned, prepared with equal volume water, 1 cup	72	12	Tr	2	Tr	0	2	822
Sweets								
3 MUSKETEERS, 1.81 oz bar	212	39	1	7	3	6	2	99
ALMOND JOY, 1.76 oz package	235	29	2	13	9	2	2	70
BABY RUTH, 0.75 oz bar	97	13	1	5	3	Tr	1	45
BUTTERFINGER, fun size bar	100	15	Tr	4	2	0	1	45
Caramels, 1 piece	39	8	Tr	1	1	1	Tr	25
Frostings, chocolate, creamy, ready-to-eat, 2 tbsp	163	26	Tr	7	2	0	Tr	75
Frozen yogurts, chocolate, 1 cup	221	38	4	6	4	23	5	110
Fruit and juice bars, 2.5 fl oz bar	63	16	1	Tr	0	0	1	3
GOOBERS, 1 serving	210	20	3	14	5	4	6	17
Gumdrops, 10 gummy bears	87	22	Tr	0	0	0	0	10
Hard candies, 1 piece	24	6	0	Tr	0	0	0	2
Honey, 1 tbsp	64	17	Tr	0	0	0	Tr	1
Ice creams, chocolate, ½ cup	143	19	1	7	4	22	3	50
Ice creams, vanilla, ½ cup	145	17	1	8	5	32	3	58
Jams and preserves, 1 tbsp	56	14	Tr	Tr	Tr	0	Tr	6
Jellies, 1 serving	56	15	Tr	Tr	Tr	0	Tr	6
Jellybeans, 10 pieces, 1 oz each	105	26	Tr	Tr	0	0	0	14
KIT KAT BIG KAT, 1.94 oz bar	286	35	1	15	10	5	3	35
KRACKEL, 1.45 oz bar	210	26	1	11	7	5	3	80
M&M's, plain, 1.69 oz package	236	34	1	10	6	7	2	29

Food, portion	Calories	Total Carb (g)	Fiber (g)	Total Fat (g)	Sat Fat (g)	Chol (mg)	Protein (g)	Sodium (mg)
M&M's, with peanuts, 1.67 oz package	243	28	2	12	5	4	4	23
Marshmallows, 1 regular	23	6	Tr	Tr	Tr	0	Tr	6
Milk chocolate, 10 kisses	246	27	2	14	7	11	4	36
MILKY WAY, 1.9 oz bar	228	39	1	9	4	8	2	130
Molasses, 1 tbsp	58	15	0	Tr	Tr	0	0	7
MR. GOODBAR, 1.75 oz bar	264	27	2	16	7	5	5	20
Nougat, 1 piece	56	13	Tr	Tr	Tr	0	Tr	5
OH HENRY!, 1 bar	120	17	1	6	2	2	2	60
Pie fillings, canned, cherry, 1 can	684	167	4	Tr	Tr	0	2	107
Puddings, chocolate, ready-to-eat, 5 oz	197	33	1	6	1	4	4	183
Puddings, rice, ready-to-eat, 5 oz	231	31	Tr	11	2	1	3	121
Puddings, tapioca, ready-to-eat, 5 oz	169	28	Tr	5	1	1	3	226
RAISINETS, 1 package	185	32	2	7	3	2	2	16
REESE'S NUTRAGEOUS, 2 bars	176	18	1	11	3	1	4	48
REESE'S Peanut Butter Cups, 1.6 oz package	232	25	2	14	5	3	5	141
Sherbet, orange, 1 bar, 2.75 fl oz	95	20	2	1	1	0	1	30
SKITTLES, 2 oz package	231	52	0	2	Tr	0	Tr	9
SNICKERS, 2 oz bar	273	34	1	14	5	7	5	152
SPECIAL DARK, 1.45 oz bar	218	24	3	13	0	2	2	2
Sugars, granulated, 1 tsp	16	4	0	0	0	0	0	na
Syrups, chocolate, fudge-type, 2 tbsp	133	24	1	3	2	1	2	131
Syrups, table blends, pancake, 1 tbsp	47	12	Tr	0	0	0	0	16
Toppings, strawberry, 2 tbsp	107	28	Tr	Tr	Tr	0	Tr	9
TWIX, 2.06 oz package	289	38	1	14	5	3	3	112
TWIZZLERS Strawberry Twists, 4 pieces	133	30	0	1	0	0	1	109
YORK Peppermint Pattie, 1 patty, 1.5 oz	165	35	1	3	2	Tr	1	12

Food, portion	Calories	Total Carb (g)	Fiber (g)	Total Fat (g)	Sat Fat (g)	Chol (mg)	Protein (g)	Sodium (mg)
Vegetables and Vegetable Products								
Artichoke, boiled, with salt, 1 artichoke	60	13	6	Tr	Tr	0	4	397
Asparagus, frozen, boiled, with salt, 1 cup	32	3	3	1	Tr	0	5	432
Bamboo shoots, boiled, drained, 1 cup	14	2	1	Tr	Tr	0	2	5
Beans, lima, canned, ½ cup	88	17	4	Tr	Tr	0	5	312
Beans, snap, green, boiled, drained, 1 cup	44	10	4	Tr	Tr	0	2	1
Beans, snap, yellow, boiled, drained, 1 cup	44	10	4	Tr	Tr	0	2	4
Beet greens, raw, 1 cup	8	2	1	Tr	Tr	0	1	86
Beets, sliced, boiled, drained, ½ cup	37	8	2	Tr	Tr	0	1	65
Broccoli, chopped, boiled, drained, ½ cup	27	6	3	Tr	Tr	0	2	32
Brussels sprouts, boiled, drained, 1 sprout	8	1	1	Tr	Tr	0	1	4
Cabbage, napa, cooked, 1 cup	13	2	na	Tr	0	0	1	12
Cabbage (pak-choi), boiled, drained, 1 cup	20	3	2	Tr	Tr	0	3	58
Carrot juice, canned, 1 cup	94	22	2	Tr	Tr	0	2	68
Carrots, baby, raw, 1 medium	4	1	Tr	Tr	Tr	0	Tr	8
Carrots, raw, 1 medium	25	6	2	Tr	Tr	0	1	42
Catsup, 1 tbsp	14	4	Tr	Tr	Tr	0	Tr	167
Cauliflower, boiled, drained, ½ cup	14	3	2	Tr	Tr	0	1	9
Celery, diced, raw, 1 cup	17	4	2	Tr	Tr	0	1	96
Chard, Swiss, chopped, boiled, drained, 1 cup	35	7	4	Tr	Tr	0	3	313
Coleslaw, home-prepared, ½ cup	41	7	1	2	Tr	5	1	14
Collards, chopped, boiled, drained, 1 cup	49	9	5	1	Tr	0	4	30
Corn, sweet, yellow, canned, cream style, 1 cup	184	46	3	1	Tr	0	4	8
Corn, sweet, yellow, raw, 1 ear	123	27	4	2	Tr	0	5	21
Cucumber, sliced, peeled, 1 cup	14	3	1	Tr	Tr	0	1	2
Eggplant, boiled, drained, 1 cup	35	9	2	Tr	Tr	0	1	1

Food, portion	Calories	Total Carb (g)	Fiber (g)	Total Fat (g)	Sat Fat (g)	Chol (mg)	Protein (g)	Sodium (mg)
Garlic, raw, 1 clove	4	1	Tr	Tr	Tr	0	Tr	1
Kale, boiled, drained, 1 cup	36	7	3	1	Tr	0	2	30
Leeks (bulb and lower leaf), raw, 1 leek	54	13	2	Tr	Tr	0	1	18
Lettuce, cos or romaine, 1 inner leaf	2	Tr	Tr	Tr	Tr	0	Tr	1
Lettuce, green leaf, 1 leaf	2	Tr	Tr	Tr	Tr	0	Tr	3
Mung beans, sprouted, stir-fried, 1 cup	62	13	2	Tr	Tr	0	5	11
Mushrooms, canned, drained, 1 medium	3	1	Tr	Tr	Tr	0	Tr	51
Mushrooms, enoki, raw, 1 medium	1	Tr	Tr	Tr	Tr	0	Tr	Tr
Mushrooms, shiitake, dried, 1 mushroom	11	3	Tr	Tr	Tr	0	Tr	Tr
Mustard greens, boiled, drained, 1 cup	21	3	3	Tr	Tr	0	3	22
Okra, sliced, boiled, drained, ½ cup	18	4	2	Tr	Tr	0	1	5
Onion rings, breaded, frozen, heated in oven, 10 rings, 2–3″ dia	244	23	1	16	5	0	3	225
Onions, boiled, drained, 1 cup	92	21	3	Tr	Tr	0	3	6
Onions, green, tops only, 1 stalk	4	1	Tr	Tr	Tr	0	Tr	Tr
Onions, raw, 1 tbsp, chopped	4	1	Tr	Tr	Tr	0	Tr	Tr
Onions, raw, 2½″ dia	46	11	2	Tr	Tr	0	1	3
Onions, raw, 1 slice, thin	4	1	Tr	Tr	Tr	0	Tr	Tr
Peas and carrots, frozen, boiled, drained, ½ cup	38	8	2	Tr	Tr	0	2	54
Peas, boiled, drained, 1 cup	67	11	4	Tr	Tr	0	5	6
Peas, green, boiled, drained, 1 cup	134	25	9	Tr	Tr	0	9	5
Peas, green, canned, seasoned, 1 cup	114	21	5	1	Tr	0	7	577
Pepper, serrano, raw, 1 pepper	2	Tr	Tr	Tr	Tr	0	Tr	1
Peppers, hot chili, green, raw, 1 pepper	18	4	1	Tr	Tr	0	1	3
Peppers, hot chili, red, raw, 1 pepper	19	4	1	Tr	Tr	0	1	4
Peppers, jalapeno, raw, 1 pepper	4	1	Tr	Tr	Tr	0	Tr	Tr

Food, portion	Calories	Total Carb (g)	Fiber (g)	Total Fat (g)	Sat Fat (g)	Chol (mg)	Protein (g)	Sodium (mg)
Vegetables and Vegetable Products *(cont.)*								
Peppers, sweet, green, raw, 1 pepper	24	6	2	Tr	Tr	0	1	4
Peppers, sweet, red, raw, 1 pepper	31	7	2	Tr	Tr	0	1	2
Peppers, sweet, yellow, raw, 1 pepper	50	12	2	Tr	Tr	0	2	4
Pickle, sour, 1 slice	1	Tr	Tr	Tr	Tr	0	Tr	85
Pickle, sweet, 1 Midget Gherkin	7	2	Tr	Tr	Tr	0	Tr	56
Pickle, sweet, 1 slice	8	2	Tr	Tr	Tr	0	Tr	66
Pickle relish, hot dog, 1 tbsp	14	4	Tr	Tr	Tr	0	Tr	164
Pickle relish, sweet, 1 tbsp	20	5	Tr	Tr	Tr	0	Tr	122
Potato, baked, flesh and skin, 1 medium, 2¼" to 3¼" dia	161	37	4	Tr	Tr	0	4	17
Potato salad, home-prepared, 1 cup	358	28	3	21	4	170	7	1323
Potatoes, au gratin, home-prepared from recipe using butter, 1 cup	323	28	4	19	12	56	12	1061
Potatoes, boiled, cooked without skin, with salt, 1 medium	144	33	3	Tr	Tr	0	3	402
Potatoes, french fried, frozen, heated in oven, with salt, 10 strips	100	16	2	4	1	0	2	133
Potatoes, hash browns, 1 cup	413	55	5	20	2	0	5	534
Potatoes, mashed, prepared from flakes, whole milk and butter, 1 cup	204	23	2	11	6	29	4	344
Potatoes, scalloped, with butter, 1 cup	211	26	5	9	6	29	7	821
Rutabagas, boiled, drained, 1 cup	66	15	3	Tr	Tr	0	2	34
Sauerkraut, canned, 1 cup	27	6	4	Tr	Tr	0	1	939
Spinach, canned, 1 cup	44	7	5	1	Tr	0	5	176
Spinach, frozen, chopped or leaf, boiled, drained, ½ cup	30	5	4	Tr	Tr	0	4	92
Squash, summer, crookneck and straightneck, sliced, boiled, drained, 1 cup	48	11	3	Tr	Tr	0	2	12

Food, portion	Calories	Total Carb (g)	Fiber (g)	Total Fat (g)	Sat Fat (g)	Chol (mg)	Protein (g)	Sodium (mg)
Sweet potato, baked in skin, 2″ dia×5″ long	103	24	4	Tr	Tr	0	2	41
Tomatillos, raw, 1 medium	11	2	1	Tr	Tr	0	Tr	Tr
Tomatoes, green, 1 medium	28	6	1	Tr	Tr	0	1	16
Tomatoes, red, canned, stewed, 1 cup	66	16	3	Tr	Tr	0	2	564
Tomatoes, red, canned, whole, 1 medium	21	5	1	Tr	Tr	0	1	11
Tomatoes, red, cooked, 1 cup	43	10	2	Tr	Tr	0	2	26
Tomatoes, red, 1 cup, chopped or sliced	32	7	2	Tr	Tr	0	2	9
Tomatoes, red, 1 cherry	4	1	Tr	Tr	Tr	0	Tr	2
Tomato juice, canned, 1 fl oz	5	1	Tr	Tr	Tr	0	Tr	3
Tomato paste, salt added, 1.6 oz can	139	32	8	1	Tr	0	7	1343
Tomato sauce, canned, with mushrooms, 1 cup	86	21	4	Tr	Tr	0	4	1107
Tomato sauce, canned, with onions, green peppers, and celery, 1 cup	103	22	4	2	Tr	0	2	1365
Tomatoes, sun-dried, 1 cup	139	30	7	2	Tr	0	8	1131
Turnip greens and turnips, frozen, boiled, drained, 1 cup	34	5	3	Tr	Tr	0	3	24
Vegetable juice cocktail, canned, 1 cup	46	11	2	Tr	Tr	0	2	653
Vegetables, mixed, canned, drained, 1 cup	80	15	5	Tr	Tr	0	4	243
Wasabi, root, raw, 1 cup, sliced	142	31	10	1	0	0	6	22
Waterchestnuts (matai), sliced, raw, ½ cup	60	15	2	Tr	Tr	0	1	9
Yam, cubed, boiled or baked, 1 cup	158	38	5	Tr	Tr	0	2	11
Zucchini, baby, raw, 1 medium	2	Tr	Tr	Tr	Tr	0	Tr	Tr
Zucchini, includes skin, frozen, boiled, drained, 1 cup	38	8	3	Tr	Tr	0	3	4

enjoy
diabetic recipes

Once you dig into these delicious recipes, you'll be amazed that dishes so good for you could be so scrumptious. Each recipe comes with the nutritional information you need to determine how the food will affect your blood sugar as well as how it will fit your calorie, fat, and sodium goals. The nutritionals can also help you mix and match foods within a meal and throughout your day so your overall diet brings you better health and tighter control. Keep in mind that the nutritional analysis for each recipe is based on a single serving, does not include garnishes or optional ingredients, and, when a range is given for an ingredient, reflects the lesser amount. Meats were trimmed of all visible fat, and cooked rice and noodles were prepared without added salt and fat.

breakfast & brunch

rice bran buttermilk pancakes

nutrients per serving:

1 pancake
Calories: 99
Carbohydrate: 18 g
Dietary Fiber: 2 g
Total Fat: 2 g
Calories From Fat: 18%
Saturated Fat: <1g
Cholesterol: 1 mg
Sodium: 119 mg
Protein: 4 g

Exchanges: 1 Starch

- 1 cup rice flour or all-purpose flour
- ¾ cup rice bran
- 1 tablespoon sugar
- 1 teaspoon baking powder
- ½ teaspoon baking soda
- 1¼ cups low-fat buttermilk
- 3 egg whites, beaten
  Vegetable cooking spray
  Fresh fruit, reduced-calorie syrup or reduced-calorie margarine (optional)

Sift together flour, bran, sugar, baking powder and baking soda in large bowl. Combine buttermilk and egg whites in small bowl; add to flour mixture. Stir until smooth. Pour ¼ cup batter onto hot griddle coated with cooking spray. Cook over medium heat until bubbles form on top and underside is lightly browned. Turn to brown other side. Serve with fresh fruit, syrup or margarine. *Makes about 10 (4-inch) pancakes*

Hint: For Cinnamon Pancakes, add 1 teaspoon ground cinnamon to dry ingredients.

Favorite recipe from *USA Rice Federation*

frittata primavera

nutrients per serving:

1 frittata wedge
(¼ of total recipe)
Calories: 112
Carbohydrate: 14 g
Dietary Fiber: 3 g
Total Fat: 3 g
Calories From Fat: 24%
Saturated Fat: 1 g
Cholesterol: 0 mg
Sodium: 145 mg
Protein: 8 g

Exchanges: 1 Starch, 1 Lean Meat

- 1 medium onion, chopped
- 1 medium red or green bell pepper, cut into strips
- 1 medium potato, peeled and grated (about 1 cup)
- 1 cup coarsely chopped broccoli
- 1 teaspoon dried oregano leaves, crushed
- ⅛ teaspoon ground black pepper
- 1 tablespoon FLEISCHMANN'S® Original Margarine
- 1 (8-ounce) container EGG BEATERS®

In 10-inch nonstick skillet or omelet pan, cook and stir onion, bell pepper, potato, broccoli, oregano and black pepper in margarine until vegetables are tender-crisp. In small bowl, with electric mixer at high speed, beat Egg Beaters® for 2 minutes until light and fluffy; pour over vegetables. Cover and cook over medium heat for 5 to 7 minutes until eggs are set. Serve from pan or carefully invert onto warm serving plate. Cut into wedges. Serve immediately. *Makes 4 servings*

rice bran buttermilk pancakes

mini vegetable quiches

nutrients per serving:

1 quiche
Calories: 115
Carbohydrate: 14 g
Dietary Fiber: 1 g
Total Fat: 4 g
Calories From Fat: 30%
Saturated Fat: 1 g
Cholesterol: 1 mg
Sodium: 184 mg
Protein: 6 g

Exchanges: ½ Starch, 2 Vegetable, ½ Fat

2 cups cut-up vegetables (bell peppers, broccoli, zucchini and/or carrots)
2 tablespoons chopped green onions
2 tablespoons FLEISCHMANN'S® Original Margarine
4 (8-inch) flour tortillas, each cut into 8 triangles
1 cup EGG BEATERS®
1 cup fat-free (skim) milk
½ teaspoon dried basil leaves

In medium nonstick skillet, over medium-high heat, sauté vegetables and green onions in margarine until tender.

Arrange 4 tortilla pieces in each of 8 (6-ounce) greased custard cups or ramekins, placing points of tortilla pieces at center of bottom of each cup and pressing lightly to form shape of cup. Divide vegetable mixture evenly among cups. In small bowl, combine Egg Beaters®, milk and basil. Pour evenly over vegetable mixture. Place cups on baking sheet. Bake at 375°F for 20 to 25 minutes or until puffed and knife inserted into centers comes out clean. Let stand 5 minutes before serving.   *Makes 8 servings*

french toast sticks

nutrients per serving:

4 sticks
Calories: 213
Carbohydrate: 25 g
Dietary Fiber: 1 g
Total Fat: 7 g
Calories From Fat: 32%
Saturated Fat: 1 g
Cholesterol: 1 mg
Sodium: 431 mg
Protein: 10 g

Exchanges: 1½ Starch, 1 Lean Meat, 1 Fat

1 cup EGG BEATERS®
⅓ cup fat-free (skim) milk
1 teaspoon ground cinnamon
1 teaspoon vanilla extract
2 tablespoons FLEISCHMANN'S® Original Margarine, divided
16 (4×1×1-inch) sticks day-old white bread
Powdered sugar, optional
Maple-flavored syrup, optional

In shallow bowl, combine Egg Beaters®, milk, cinnamon and vanilla.

In large nonstick griddle or skillet, over medium-high heat, melt 2 teaspoons margarine. Dip bread sticks in egg mixture to coat; transfer to griddle. Cook sticks on each side until golden, adding remaining margarine as needed. Dust lightly with powdered sugar and serve with syrup, if desired.   *Makes 4 servings*

Prep Time: 15 minutes
Cook Time: 18 minutes

mini vegetable quiches

brunch-time zucchini-date bread

nutrients per serving:

1 slice
(1/16 of loaf) with about 1 tablespoon spread

Calories: 124
Carbohydrate: 24 g
Dietary Fiber: 2 g
Total Fat: 1 g
Calories From Fat: 7%
Saturated Fat: <1 g
Cholesterol: 27 mg
Sodium: 260 mg
Protein: 5 g

Exchanges: 1 1/2 Starch

Bread
1 cup chopped pitted dates
1 cup water
1 cup whole wheat flour
1 cup all-purpose flour
2 tablespoons granulated sugar
1 teaspoon baking powder
1/2 teaspoon baking soda
1/2 teaspoon salt
1/2 teaspoon ground cinnamon
1/4 teaspoon ground cloves
2 eggs
1 cup shredded zucchini, pressed dry with paper towels

Cream Cheese Spread
1 package (8 ounces) fat-free cream cheese
1/4 cup powdered sugar
1 tablespoon vanilla
1/8 teaspoon ground cinnamon
Dash ground cloves

1. Preheat oven to 350°F. Spray 8×4×2-inch loaf pan with nonstick cooking spray.

2. For bread, combine dates and water in small saucepan. Bring to a boil over medium-high heat. Remove from heat; let stand 15 minutes.

3. Combine flours, granulated sugar, baking powder, baking soda, salt, cinnamon and 1/4 teaspoon ground cloves in large bowl. Beat eggs in medium bowl; stir in date mixture and zucchini. Stir egg mixture into flour mixture just until dry ingredients are moistened. Pour batter evenly into prepared pan. Bake 30 to 35 minutes or until toothpick inserted into center comes out clean. Cool 5 minutes. Remove from pan. Cool completely on wire rack.

4. Meanwhile, prepare cream cheese spread. Combine cream cheese, powdered sugar, vanilla, cinnamon and dash ground cloves in small bowl. Beat until smooth. Cover and refrigerate until ready to use.

5. Cut bread into 16 slices. Serve with cream cheese spread. *Makes 16 servings*

brunch-time zucchini-date bread

western omelet

½ **cup finely chopped red or green bell pepper**
⅓ **cup cubed cooked potato**
2 **slices turkey bacon, diced**
¼ **teaspoon dried oregano leaves**
2 **teaspoons FLEISCHMANN'S® Original Margarine, divided**
1 **cup EGG BEATERS®**
  Fresh oregano sprig, for garnish

In 8-inch nonstick skillet, over medium heat, sauté bell pepper, potato, turkey bacon and dried oregano in 1 teaspoon margarine until tender. Remove from skillet; keep warm.

In same skillet, over medium heat, melt remaining margarine. Pour Egg Beaters® into skillet. Cook, lifting edges to allow uncooked portion to flow underneath. When almost set, spoon vegetable mixture over half of omelet. Fold other half over vegetable mixture; slide onto serving plate. Garnish with fresh oregano.   *Makes 2 servings*

Note: For frittata, sauté vegetables, turkey bacon and dried oregano in 2 teaspoons margarine. Pour Egg Beaters® evenly into skillet over vegetable mixture. Cook without stirring for 4 to 5 minutes or until cooked on bottom and almost set on top. Carefully turn frittata; cook for 1 to 2 minutes more or until done. Slide onto serving platter; cut into wedges to serve.

Prep Time: 15 minutes
Cook Time: 10 minutes

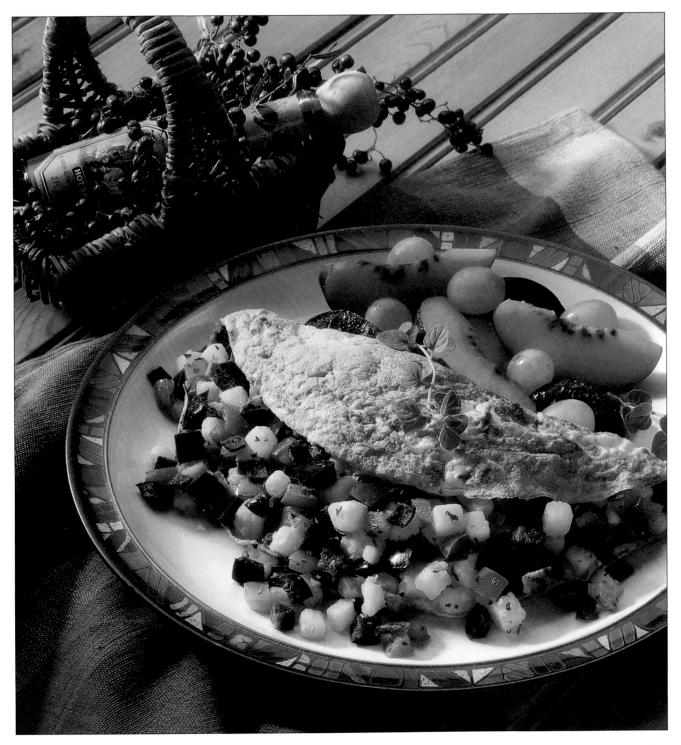

western omelet

blueberry-sour cream corn muffins

nutrients per serving:

1 muffin with about
1 tablespoon spread

Calories: 150
Carbohydrate: 23 g
Dietary Fiber: 1 g
Total Fat: 4 g
Calories From Fat: 24%
Saturated Fat: 3 g
Cholesterol: 29 mg
Sodium: 252 mg
Protein: 5 g

Exchanges: 1 Starch,
½ Fruit, 1 Fat

1 cup all-purpose flour
¾ cup cornmeal
2 teaspoons baking powder
½ teaspoon baking soda
¼ teaspoon salt
1 egg, beaten
1 cup reduced-fat sour cream
⅓ cup frozen unsweetened apple juice concentrate, thawed
1½ cups fresh or frozen (not thawed) blueberries
⅔ cup reduced-fat whipped cream cheese
2 tablespoons no-sugar-added blueberry fruit spread

1. Preheat oven to 400°F. Spray 12 medium-size muffin cups with nonstick cooking spray, or line with paper liners; set aside.

2. Combine flour, cornmeal, baking powder, baking soda and salt in medium bowl. Add combined egg, sour cream and apple juice concentrate; mix just until dry ingredients are moistened. Gently stir in blueberries.

3. Spoon batter into prepared muffin cups, filling each cup ¾ full. Bake 18 to 20 minutes or until golden brown. Let stand in pan on wire rack 5 minutes. Remove from pan; cool slightly. Combine cream cheese and fruit spread in small serving bowl; serve with warm muffins.

Makes 1 dozen muffins

blueberry-sour cream corn muffins

farmstand frittata

Nonstick cooking spray
½ **cup chopped onion**
1 **medium red bell pepper, seeded and cut into thin strips**
1 **cup broccoli florets, blanched and drained**
1 **cup cooked, quartered unpeeled red potatoes**
1 **cup cholesterol-free egg substitute**
6 **egg whites**
1 **tablespoon chopped fresh parsley**
½ **teaspoon salt**
¼ **teaspoon black pepper**
½ **cup (2 ounces) shredded reduced-fat Cheddar cheese**

1. Spray large nonstick ovenproof skillet with cooking spray; heat over medium heat until hot. Add onion and bell pepper; cook and stir 3 minutes or until crisp-tender.

2. Add broccoli and potatoes; cook and stir 1 to 2 minutes or until heated through.

3. Whisk together egg substitute, egg whites, parsley, salt and black pepper in medium bowl.

4. Spread vegetables into even layer in skillet. Pour egg white mixture over vegetables; cover and cook over medium heat 10 to 12 minutes or until egg mixture is set.

5. Meanwhile, preheat broiler. Top frittata with cheese. Broil 4 inches from heat 1 minute or until cheese is melted. Cut into 4 wedges to serve.   *Makes 4 servings*

farmstand frittata

ham and cheese corn muffins

nutrients per serving:

1 muffin (without honey-flavored butter)
Calories: 150
Carbohydrate: 18 g
Dietary Fiber: 2 g
Total Fat: 6 g
Calories From Fat: 35%
Saturated Fat: 2 g
Cholesterol: 33 mg
Sodium: 411 mg
Protein: 6 g

Exchanges: 1 Starch, 1 Lean Meat, ½ Fat

1 package (about 8 ounces) corn muffin mix
½ cup chopped deli ham
½ cup (2 ounces) shredded Swiss cheese
⅓ cup reduced-fat (2%) milk
1 egg
1 tablespoon Dijon mustard

1. Preheat oven to 400°F. Combine muffin mix, ham and cheese in medium bowl.

2. Combine milk, egg and mustard in 1-cup glass measure. Stir milk mixture into dry ingredients; mix just until moistened.

3. Fill 9 paper-cup-lined 2¾-inch muffin cups ⅔ full with batter.

4. Bake 18 to 20 minutes or until light golden brown. Remove muffin pan to cooling rack. Let stand 5 minutes. Serve warm. *Makes 9 muffins*

Serving Suggestion: For added flavor, serve Ham and Cheese Corn Muffins with honey-flavored butter. To prepare, stir together equal amounts of honey and softened butter.

potato & onion frittata

nutrients per serving:

1 frittata wedge (½ of total recipe)
Calories: 179
Carbohydrate: 19 g
Dietary Fiber: 2 g
Total Fat: 5 g
Calories From Fat: 25%
Saturated Fat: 1 g
Cholesterol: 0 mg
Sodium: 276 mg
Protein: 14 g

Exchanges: 1 Starch, 1 Vegetable, ½ Lean Meat, ½ Fat

1 small baking potato, peeled, halved and sliced ⅛ inch thick (about ½ cup)
¼ cup chopped onion
1 clove garlic, minced
Dash ground black pepper
1 tablespoon FLEISCHMANN'S® Original Margarine
1 cup EGG BEATERS®

In 8-inch nonstick skillet, over medium-high heat, sauté potato, onion, garlic and pepper in margarine until tender. Pour Egg Beaters® evenly into skillet over potato mixture. Cook, without stirring, for 5 to 6 minutes or until cooked on bottom and almost set on top. Carefully turn frittata; cook for 1 to 2 minutes more or until done. Slide onto serving platter; cut into wedges to serve. *Makes 2 servings*

Prep Time: 5 minutes
Cook Time: 15 minutes

ham and cheese corn muffins

eggs primavera

nutrients per serving:

1 bread bowl with about 1 cup egg mixture (¼ of total recipe)

Calories: 201
Carbohydrate: 23 g
Dietary Fiber: 4 g
Total Fat: 6 g
Calories From Fat: 26%
Saturated Fat: 2 g
Cholesterol: 114 mg
Sodium: 336 mg
Protein: 14 g

Exchanges: 1 Starch, 1½ Vegetable, 1½ Lean Meat

4 small round loaves (4 inches each) whole wheat bread
  Nonstick cooking spray
1½ cups chopped onions
 ¾ cup chopped yellow summer squash
 ¾ cup chopped zucchini
 ½ cup chopped red bell pepper
 2 ounces snow peas, trimmed and cut diagonally into thirds
 ¼ cup finely chopped fresh parsley
1½ teaspoons finely chopped fresh thyme *or* ¾ teaspoon dried thyme leaves
 1 teaspoon finely chopped fresh rosemary *or* ½ teaspoon dried rosemary leaves, crushed
 2 whole eggs
 4 egg whites
 ¼ teaspoon black pepper
 ½ cup (2 ounces) shredded reduced-fat Swiss cheese

1. Preheat oven to 350°F. Slice top off each loaf of bread. Carefully hollow out each loaf, leaving sides and bottom ½ inch thick. Reserve centers for another use. Place loaves and tops, cut sides up, on baking sheet. Spray all surfaces of bread with cooking spray; bake 15 minutes or until well toasted.

2. Spray large nonstick skillet with cooking spray and heat over medium heat until hot. Add onions; cook and stir 3 minutes or until soft. Add yellow squash, zucchini and bell pepper; cook and stir 3 minutes or until crisp-tender. Add snow peas and herbs; cook and stir 1 minute.

3. Whisk eggs, egg whites and black pepper in small bowl until blended. Add to vegetable mixture; gently stir until eggs begin to set. Sprinkle cheese over top; gently stir until cheese melts and eggs are set but not dry.

4. Fill each bread bowl with ¼ of egg mixture, about 1 cup. Place tops back on bread bowls before serving. Garnish, if desired. *Makes 4 servings*

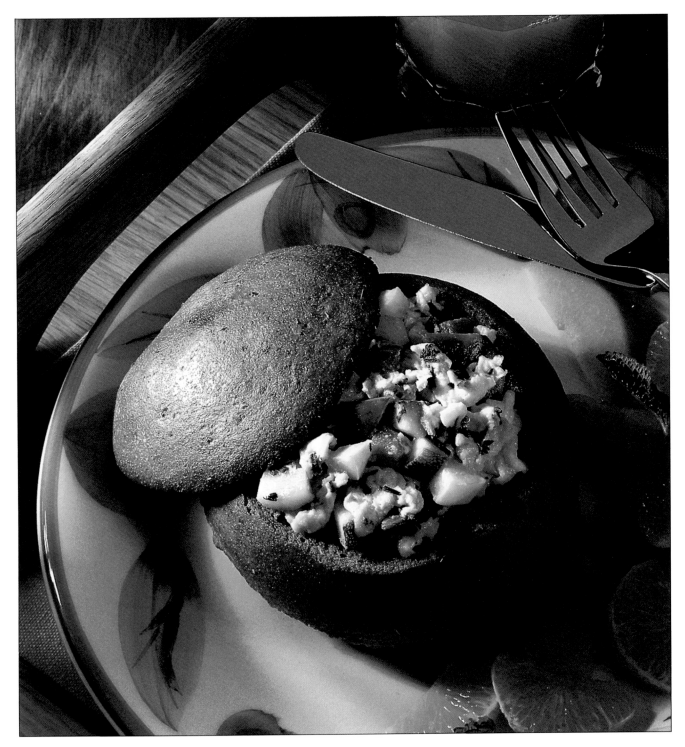

eggs primavera

strawberry oat mini muffins

nutrients per serving:

3 mini muffins

Calories: 135
Carbohydrate: 23 g
Dietary Fiber: 2 g
Total Fat: 3 g
Calories From Fat: 21%
Saturated Fat: <1 g
Cholesterol: 1 mg
Sodium: 310 mg
Protein: 4 g

Exchanges: 1½ Starch, ½ Fat

1 cup all-purpose flour
¾ cup uncooked oat bran cereal
2½ teaspoons baking powder
½ teaspoon baking soda
⅛ teaspoon salt
¾ cup buttermilk
⅓ cup frozen apple juice concentrate, thawed
⅓ cup unsweetened applesauce
½ teaspoon vanilla
¾ cup diced strawberries
¼ cup chopped pecans

1. Preheat oven to 400°F. Spray 24 miniature muffin cups with nonstick cooking spray.

2. Combine flour, oat bran, baking powder, baking soda and salt in medium bowl. Whisk together buttermilk, apple juice concentrate, applesauce and vanilla in small bowl.

3. Stir buttermilk mixture into flour mixture just until dry ingredients are almost moistened. Fold strawberries and pecans into batter. *Do not overmix.*

4. Spoon batter into muffin cups. Bake 17 to 18 minutes or until lightly browned and toothpick inserted into centers comes out clean. Let cool in pan 5 minutes; remove to wire racks. Serve warm or cool completely.   *Makes 2 dozen mini muffins*

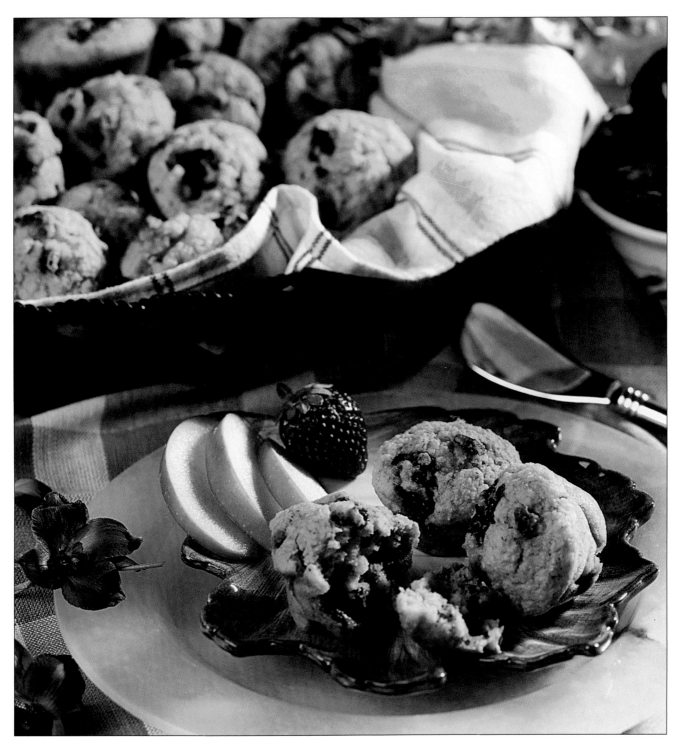

strawberry oat mini muffins

nutrients per serving:

1 cup strata
Calories: 155
Carbohydrate: 20 g
Dietary Fiber: 3 g
Total Fat: 2 g
Calories From Fat: 12%
Saturated Fat: 1 g
Cholesterol: 8 mg
Sodium: 642 mg
Protein: 15 g

Exchanges: 1½ Starch, 2 Lean Meat

brunch strata

2 cups cholesterol-free egg substitute *or* 8 eggs
1 can (10¾ ounces) reduced-fat condensed cream of celery soup, undiluted
1 cup fat-free (skim) milk
1 can (4 ounces) sliced mushrooms, drained (optional)
¼ cup sliced green onions
1 teaspoon dry mustard
½ teaspoon salt (optional)
¼ teaspoon black pepper
6 slices reduced-fat white bread, cut into 1-inch cubes
4 links reduced-fat precooked breakfast sausage, thinly sliced

1. Preheat oven to 350°F. Spray 2-quart baking dish with nonstick cooking spray; set aside.

2. Combine egg substitute, soup, milk, mushrooms, if desired, green onions, mustard, salt, if desired, and pepper in medium bowl; mix well.

3. Combine bread cubes, sausage and soup mixture in prepared baking dish; toss to coat. Bake 35 to 40 minutes or until set. Garnish as desired.   *Makes 6 servings*

tip

Look for the words "light," "lite," "reduced-fat" or "fat-free" when you're shopping for the ingredients in this recipe.

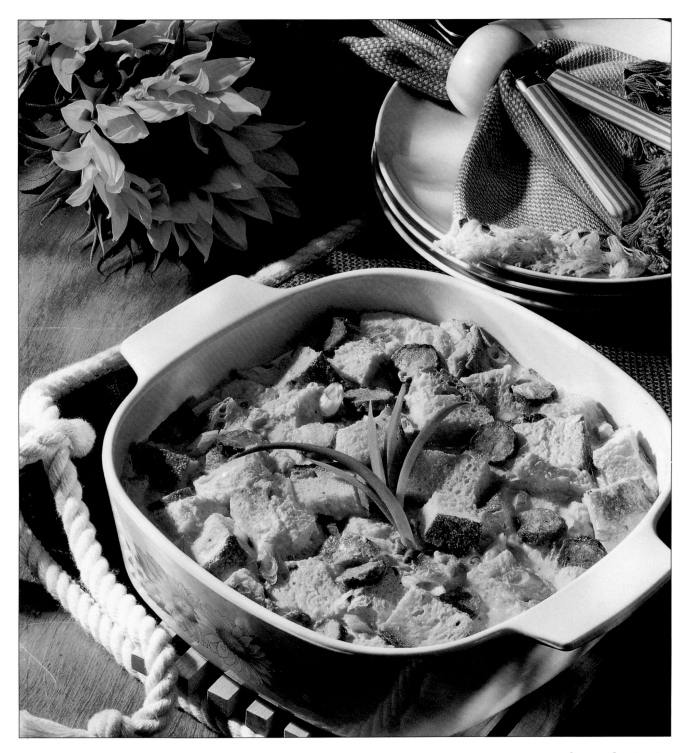

brunch strata

scrambled egg burritos

nutrients per serving:

1 burrito with 1 tablespoon plus 1 teaspoon salsa

Calories: 186
Carbohydrate: 23 g
Dietary Fiber: 1 g
Total Fat: 4 g
Calories From Fat: 20%
Saturated Fat: 1 g
Cholesterol: 6 mg
Sodium: 423 mg
Protein: 14 g

Exchanges: 1 Starch, 1 Vegetable, 1½ Lean Meat

Nonstick cooking spray
1 medium red bell pepper, chopped
5 green onions, sliced
½ teaspoon red pepper flakes
1 cup cholesterol-free egg substitute *or* 8 egg whites
1 tablespoon chopped fresh cilantro or parsley
4 (8-inch) flour tortillas
½ cup (2 ounces) shredded low-sodium reduced-fat Monterey Jack cheese
⅓ cup salsa

1. Spray medium nonstick skillet with cooking spray. Heat over medium heat until hot. Add bell pepper, green onions and red pepper flakes; cook and stir 3 minutes or until vegetables are crisp-tender.

2. Add egg substitute to vegetables. Reduce heat to low. Cook and stir 3 minutes or until set. Sprinkle with cilantro.

3. Stack tortillas and wrap in paper towels. Microwave at HIGH 1 minute or until tortillas are hot.

4. Place ¼ egg mixture on each tortilla. Sprinkle with 2 tablespoons cheese. Fold sides over to enclose filling. Serve with salsa. *Makes 4 servings*

tip

Store the cilantro or parsley for this recipe in a tall glass in the refrigerator. Fill the glass with enough cold water to cover about 1 inch of the stems, then top the leaves with a plastic bag. Use a rubber band to attach the bag to the top of the glass.

scrambled egg burrito

spicy mexican frittata

1 fresh jalapeño pepper*
1 clove garlic
1 medium tomato, peeled, halved, quartered and seeded
½ teaspoon ground coriander
½ teaspoon chili powder
Nonstick cooking spray
½ cup chopped onion
1 cup frozen corn
6 egg whites
2 eggs
¼ cup fat-free (skim) milk
¼ teaspoon salt
¼ teaspoon black pepper
¼ cup (1 ounce) shredded part-skim farmer or mozzarella cheese

Jalapeño peppers can sting and irritate the skin. Wear rubber gloves when handling peppers and do not touch eyes. Wash hands after handling peppers.

1. Place jalapeño pepper and garlic in food processor or blender. Cover; process until finely chopped. Add tomato, coriander and chili powder. Cover; process until tomato is almost smooth.

2. Spray large skillet with cooking spray; heat over medium heat until hot. Cook and stir onion until tender. Stir in tomato mixture and corn; cook 3 to 4 minutes or until liquid is almost evaporated, stirring occasionally.

3. Combine egg whites, eggs, milk, salt and black pepper in medium bowl. Add egg mixture all at once to skillet. Cook, without stirring, 2 minutes or until eggs begin to set. Run large spoon around edge of skillet, lifting eggs for even cooking. Remove skillet from heat when eggs are almost set but surface is still moist.

4. Sprinkle with cheese. Cover; let stand 3 to 4 minutes or until surface is set and cheese is melted. Cut into 4 wedges.   *Makes 4 servings*

spicy mexican frittata

snacks & appetizers

nutrients per serving:

1 quesadilla wedge with about 1½ tablespoons pico de gallo

Calories: 79

Carbohydrate: 12 g

Dietary Fiber: 1 g

Total Fat: 2 g

Calories From Fat: 21%

Saturated Fat: 1 g

Cholesterol: 4 mg

Sodium: 223 mg

Protein: 4 g

Exchanges: 1 Starch

veggie quesadilla appetizers

10 (8-inch) flour tortillas
1 cup finely chopped broccoli
1 cup thinly sliced small mushrooms
¾ cup shredded carrots
¼ cup chopped green onions
1¼ cups (5 ounces) reduced-fat sharp Cheddar cheese
2 cups Zesty Pico de Gallo (recipe follows)

1. Brush both sides of tortillas lightly with water. Heat small nonstick skillet over medium heat until hot. Heat tortillas, one at a time, 30 seconds on each side. Divide vegetables among 5 tortillas; sprinkle evenly with cheese. Top with remaining 5 tortillas.

2. Cook quesadillas, one at a time, in large nonstick skillet or on griddle over medium heat 2 minutes on each side or until surface is crisp and cheese is melted.

3. Cut each quesadilla into 4 wedges. Serve with Zesty Pico de Gallo.

Makes 20 servings

zesty pico de gallo

2 cups chopped seeded tomatoes
1 cup chopped green onions
1 can (8 ounces) tomato sauce
½ cup minced fresh cilantro
1 to 2 tablespoons minced jalapeño peppers*
1 tablespoon fresh lime juice

*Jalapeño peppers can sting and irritate the skin. Wear rubber gloves when handling peppers and do not touch eyes. Wash hands after handling peppers.

Combine all ingredients in medium bowl. Cover and refrigerate at least 1 hour.

Makes about 4 cups

veggie quesadilla appetizer

lox and cheese mini pizzas

New York-Style Pizza Crust (page 184)
4 ounces reduced-fat cream cheese
2 tablespoons finely chopped red onion
1 tablespoon fresh lemon juice
2 teaspoons grated fresh lemon peel
1½ teaspoons olive oil
4 ounces thinly sliced lox or smoked salmon
Black pepper
1 tablespoon small capers, 2 teaspoons snipped fresh chives *or*
20 tiny sprigs fresh dill, for garnish (optional)

1. Prepare New York-Style Pizza Crust as directed through step 2. Preheat oven to 500°F. Lightly grease 2 large baking sheets; set aside.

2. Combine cream cheese, onion, lemon juice and lemon peel in small bowl; set aside.

3. Roll out dough into 10-inch log on lightly floured surface. Cut log into 20 (½-inch-thick) slices. Pat slices into 2¼- to 2½-inch discs. Place slightly apart on prepared baking sheets. Pierce discs several times with fork; brush evenly with oil. Bake, 1 sheet at a time, 6 minutes or until light golden. Transfer to wire rack to cool slightly.

4. Spoon about 1 teaspoon cream cheese mixture onto center of each warm crust. Spread over surface, leaving ¼-inch border. Cut lox into 2-inch pieces. Place over cream cheese. Sprinkle with pepper. Garnish, if desired.   *Makes 20 mini pizzas*

Note: To prepare the mini pizza crusts in advance, let the baked crusts cool completely on wire racks after being removed from the oven. Store the crusts in an airtight container at room temperature for up to one day.

continued on page 184

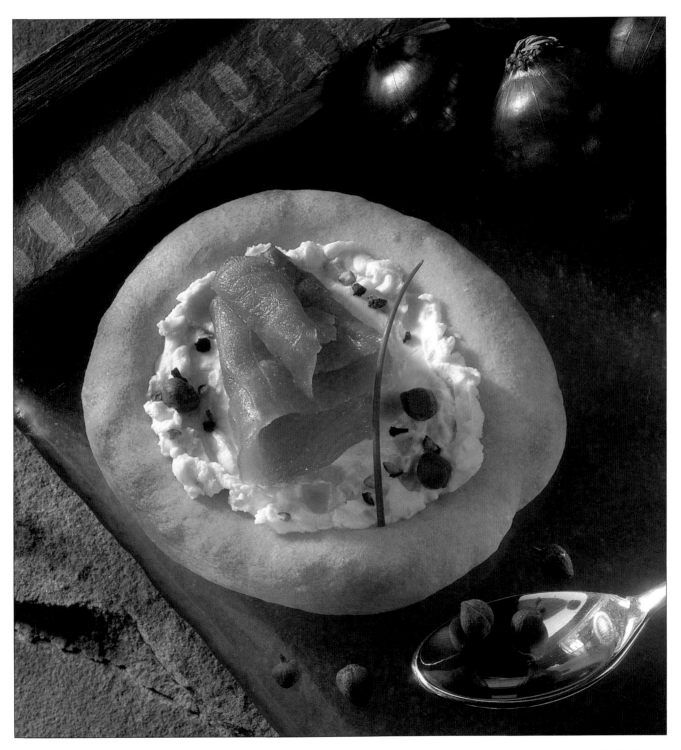

lox and cheese mini pizza

lox and cheese mini pizzas, continued

new york-style pizza crust

²⁄₃ **cup warm water (110°F to 115°F)**
1 **teaspoon sugar**
½ **(¼-ounce) package rapid-rise or active dry yeast**
1¾ **cups all-purpose or bread flour plus additional for kneading**
½ **teaspoon salt**
1 **tablespoon cornmeal (optional)**

1. Combine water and sugar in small bowl; stir to dissolve sugar. Sprinkle yeast over top; stir to combine. Let stand 5 to 10 minutes or until foamy.

2. Combine flour and salt in medium bowl. Stir in yeast mixture. Mix until mixture forms soft dough. Remove dough to lightly floured surface. Knead 5 minutes or until dough is smooth and elastic, adding additional flour, 1 tablespoon at a time, as needed. Place dough in medium bowl coated with nonstick cooking spray. Turn dough in bowl so top is coated with cooking spray; cover with towel or plastic wrap. Let rise in warm place 30 minutes or until doubled in bulk. Punch dough down; place on lightly floured surface and knead about 2 minutes or until smooth.

3. Pat dough into flat disc about 7 inches in diameter. Let rest 2 to 3 minutes. Pat and gently stretch dough from edges until dough seems to not stretch anymore. Let rest 2 to 3 minutes. Continue patting and stretching until dough is 12 to 14 inches in diameter.

4. Spray 12- to 14-inch pizza pan with nonstick cooking spray; sprinkle with cornmeal, if desired. Press dough into pan.

5. Preheat oven to 500°F. Follow directions for individual recipes, baking pizza on bottom rack of oven.

Makes 20 (2½-inch) mini pizza crusts, 1 medium-thin 12-inch crust,
1 very thin 14-inch crust, 2 (8- to 9-inch) crusts or 4 (6- to 7- inch) crusts

cheesy potato skin appetizers

⅔ **cup Zesty Pico de Gallo (page 180) or purchased salsa**
5 **potatoes (4 to 5 ounces each)**
   Butter-flavored nonstick cooking spray
4 **ounces fat-free cream cheese**
2 **tablespoons reduced-fat sour cream**
⅓ **cup (about 1.3 ounces) shredded reduced-fat sharp Cheddar cheese**
2 **tablespoons sliced ripe olives (optional)**
¼ **cup minced fresh cilantro**

1. Prepare Zesty Pico de Gallo; set aside.

2. Preheat oven to 425°F. Scrub potatoes; pierce several times with fork. Bake 45 minutes or until soft. Cool.

3. Split each potato lengthwise into halves. Scoop out potato with spoon, leaving ¼-inch-thick shell. (Reserve potato for another use, if desired.) Place potato skins on baking sheet; spray lightly with cooking spray.

4. Preheat broiler. Broil potato skins 6 inches from heat 5 minutes or until lightly browned and crisp.

5. Preheat oven to 350°F. Combine cream cheese and sour cream in small bowl; stir until well blended. Divide evenly among potato skins; spread to cover. Top with Zesty Pico do Gallo, cheese and olives, if desired. Bake 15 minutes or until heated through. Sprinkle with cilantro.

Makes 10 servings

nutrients per serving:

1 potato skin appetizer with about 1 tablespoon pico de gallo

Calories: 86
Carbohydrate: 15 g
Dietary Fiber: 3 g
Total Fat: 1 g
Calories From Fat: 10%
Saturated Fat: 1 g
Cholesterol: 4 mg
Sodium: 149 mg
Protein: 4 g

Exchanges: 1 Starch, ½ Lean Meat

portobello mushrooms sesame

4 large portobello mushrooms
2 tablespoons sweet rice wine
2 tablespoons reduced-sodium soy sauce
2 cloves garlic, minced
1 teaspoon dark sesame oil

1. Remove and discard stems from mushrooms; set caps aside. Combine remaining ingredients in small bowl.

2. Brush both sides of mushroom caps with soy sauce mixture. Grill mushrooms, top sides up, on covered grill over medium coals 3 to 4 minutes. Brush tops with soy sauce mixture and turn over; grill 2 minutes more or until mushrooms are lightly browned. Turn again and grill, basting frequently, 4 to 5 minutes or until tender when pressed with back of metal spatula. Remove mushrooms; cut diagonally into ½-inch-thick slices.

Makes 4 servings

mediterranean pita pizzas

1 cup canned cannellini beans, rinsed and drained
2 teaspoons lemon juice
2 medium cloves garlic, minced
2 (8-inch) pita bread rounds
1 teaspoon olive oil
½ cup thinly sliced radicchio or escarole lettuce (optional)
½ cup chopped seeded tomato
½ cup finely chopped red onion
¼ cup (1 ounce) crumbled feta cheese
2 tablespoons thinly sliced pitted black olives

1. Preheat oven to 450°F. Place beans in small bowl; mash lightly with fork. Stir in lemon juice and garlic.

2. Arrange pita rounds on baking sheet; brush tops with oil. Bake 6 minutes.

3. Spread bean mixture onto pita rounds to within ½ inch of edges. Arrange remaining ingredients on pitas. Bake 5 minutes or until topping is thoroughly heated and crust is crisp. Cut each pizza into 4 wedges. Serve hot.

Makes 8 servings

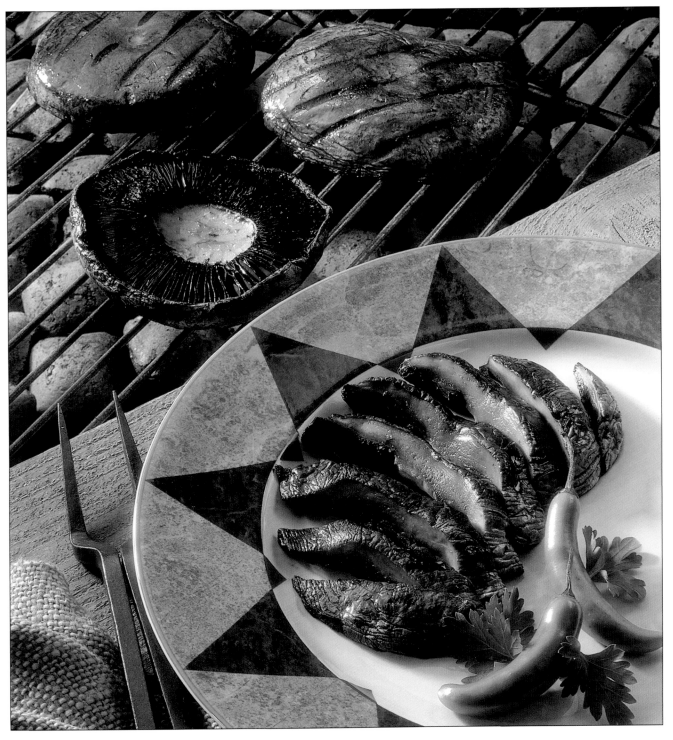

portobello mushrooms sesame

señor nacho dip

4 ounces fat-free cream cheese
½ cup (2 ounces) shredded reduced-fat Cheddar cheese
¼ cup mild or medium chunky salsa
2 teaspoons reduced-fat (2%) milk
4 ounces baked tortilla chips or assorted fresh vegetable dippers

1. Combine cream cheese and Cheddar cheese in small saucepan; cook and stir over low heat until melted. Stir in salsa and milk; heat thoroughly, stirring occasionally.

2. Transfer dip to small serving bowl. Serve with tortilla chips. Garnish with hot peppers and cilantro, if desired. *Makes 4 servings*

Olé Dip: Substitute reduced-fat Monterey Jack cheese or reduced-fat taco cheese for Cheddar cheese.

Spicy Mustard Dip: Omit tortilla chips. Substitute 2 teaspoons spicy brown mustard or honey mustard for salsa. Serve with fresh vegetable dippers or pretzels.

nutrients per serving:

about 3½ tablespoons dip with 10 tortilla chips
Calories: 181
Carbohydrate: 25 g
Dietary Fiber: 2 g
Total Fat: 4 g
Calories From Fat: 18%
Saturated Fat: 1 g
Cholesterol: 11 mg
Sodium: 629 mg
Protein: 11 g

Exchanges: 1½ Starch, 1 Lean Meat

california rolls

1 cup reduced-fat ricotta cheese
2 (11-inch) flour tortillas
1 medium tomato, thinly sliced
2 cups stemmed, washed and torn fresh spinach leaves
1 cup chopped onion
½ teaspoon dried oregano leaves
½ teaspoon dried basil leaves
1 cup alfalfa sprouts
4 ounces sliced turkey breast

Spread cheese evenly over tortillas to within ¼ inch of edges. Layer tomato, spinach, onion, oregano, basil, alfalfa sprouts and turkey over ⅔ of each tortilla. Roll up tortillas. Wrap in plastic wrap; refrigerate 1 hour. Cut each rolled tortilla crosswise into 10 slices before serving. *Makes 4 servings*

nutrients per serving:

5 rolls
Calories: 209
Carbohydrate: 28 g
Dietary Fiber: 2 g
Total Fat: 4 g
Calories From Fat: 17%
Saturated Fat: <1 g
Cholesterol: 28 mg
Sodium: 233 mg
Protein: 16 g

Exchanges: 1½ Starch, 1 Vegetable, 1½ Lean Meat

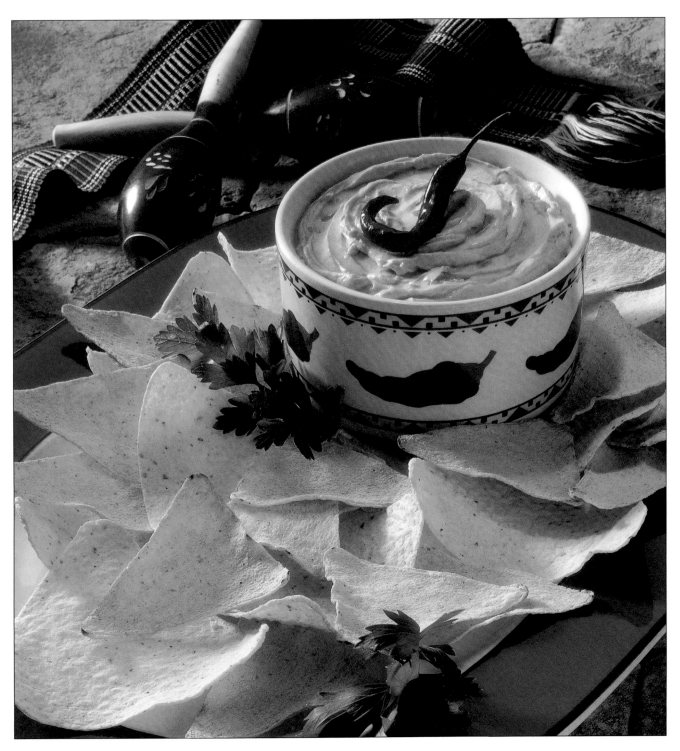

señor nacho dip

stuffed party baguette

2 medium red bell peppers
1 French bread loaf (about 14 inches long)
¼ cup plus 2 tablespoons prepared fat-free Italian dressing, divided
1 small red onion, very thinly sliced
8 large fresh basil leaves
3 ounces Swiss cheese, very thinly sliced

1. Preheat oven to 425°F. Cover large baking sheet with foil; set aside.

2. To roast bell peppers, cut peppers in half; remove stems, seeds and membranes. Place peppers, cut sides down, on prepared baking sheet. Bake 20 to 25 minutes or until skins are browned, turning occasionally.

3. Transfer peppers from baking sheet to paper bag; close bag tightly. Let stand 10 minutes or until peppers are cool enough to handle and skins are loosened. Using sharp knife, peel off skins; discard skins. Cut peppers into strips.

4. Trim ends from bread; discard. Cut loaf lengthwise in half. Remove soft insides of loaf; reserve removed bread for another use, if desired.

5. Brush ¼ cup Italian dressing evenly onto cut sides of bread. Arrange pepper strips in even layer in bottom half of loaf; top with even layer of onion. Brush onion with remaining 2 tablespoons Italian dressing; top with layer of basil and cheese. Replace bread top. Wrap loaf tightly in heavy-duty plastic wrap; refrigerate at least 2 hours or overnight.

6. When ready to serve, remove plastic wrap. Cut loaf crosswise into 1-inch slices. Secure with toothpicks and garnish, if desired. *Makes 12 servings*

stuffed party baguette

spicy orange chicken kabob appetizers

nutrients per serving:

2 kabobs

Calories: 30
Carbohydrate: 2 g
Dietary Fiber: <1 g
Total Fat: <1 g
Calories From Fat: 26%
Saturated Fat: <1 g
Cholesterol: 10 mg
Sodium: 38 mg
Protein: 4 g

Exchanges: ½ Lean Meat

    2 boneless skinless chicken breasts (4 ounces each)
    1 small red or green bell pepper
   24 small fresh button mushrooms
    ½ cup orange juice
    2 tablespoons reduced-sodium soy sauce
    1 tablespoon vegetable oil
  1½ teaspoons onion powder
    ½ teaspoon Chinese five-spice powder

1. Cut chicken and pepper each into 24 (¾-inch) square pieces. Place chicken, pepper and mushrooms in large resealable plastic food storage bag. Combine orange juice, soy sauce, oil, onion powder and five-spice powder in small bowl. Pour over chicken mixture. Close bag securely; turn to coat. Marinate in refrigerator 4 to 24 hours, turning frequently.

2. Soak 24 small wooden skewers or toothpicks in water 20 minutes. Meanwhile, preheat broiler. Coat broiler pan with nonstick cooking spray.

3. Drain chicken, pepper and mushrooms, reserving marinade. Thread 1 piece chicken, 1 piece pepper and 1 mushroom onto each skewer. Place on prepared pan. Brush with marinade; discard remaining marinade. Broil 4 inches from heat 5 to 6 minutes or until chicken is no longer pink in center. Serve immediately.   *Makes 12 servings*

snackin' cinnamon popcorn

nutrients per serving:

2 cups popcorn

Calories: 63
Carbohydrate: 13 g
Dietary Fiber: 3 g
Total Fat: 1 g
Calories From Fat: 9%
Saturated Fat: <1 g
Cholesterol: 0 mg
Sodium: 873 mg
Protein: 2 g

Exchanges: 1 Starch

    3 to 4 teaspoons brown sugar substitute
  1½ teaspoons salt
  1½ teaspoons cinnamon
    8 cups hot air-popped popcorn
      Butter-flavored nonstick cooking spray

1. Combine brown sugar substitute, salt and cinnamon in small bowl; mix well.

2. Spread hot popped popcorn onto jelly-roll pan. Coat popcorn with cooking spray; immediately sprinkle cinnamon mixture over top. Serve immediately or store in container at room temperature up to 2 days.   *Makes 4 servings*

spicy orange chicken kabob appetizers

oven-fried tex-mex onion rings

nutrients per serving:

about 8 onion rings

Calories: 111
Carbohydrate: 16 g
Dietary Fiber: 2 g
Total Fat: 4 g
Calories From Fat: 30%
Saturated Fat: 1 g
Cholesterol: 0 mg
Sodium: 188 mg
Protein: 4 g

Exchanges: 1 Starch,
½ Fat

½ cup plain dry bread crumbs
⅓ cup yellow cornmeal
1½ teaspoons chili powder
⅛ to ¼ teaspoon ground red pepper
⅛ teaspoon salt
1 tablespoon plus 1½ teaspoons margarine, melted
1 teaspoon water
2 medium onions (about 10 ounces), sliced ⅜ inch thick
2 egg whites

1. Preheat oven to 450°F. Spray large nonstick baking sheet with nonstick cooking spray; set aside.

2. Combine bread crumbs, cornmeal, chili powder, ground red pepper and salt in medium shallow dish; mix well. Stir in margarine and water.

3. Separate onion slices into rings. Place egg whites in large bowl; beat lightly. Add onions; toss lightly to coat evenly. Transfer to bread crumb mixture; toss to coat evenly. Place in single layer on prepared baking sheet. Bake 12 to 15 minutes or until onions are tender and coating is crisp. *Makes 6 servings*

rock 'n' rollers

nutrients per serving:

2 rock 'n' roller halves

Calories: 315
Carbohydrate: 41 g
Dietary Fiber: 2 g
Total Fat: 9 g
Calories From Fat: 26%
Saturated Fat: 5 g
Cholesterol: 31 mg
Sodium: 865 mg
Protein: 17 g

Exchanges: 2½ Starch,
1 Lean Meat, 1½ Fat

4 (6- to 7-inch) flour tortillas
4 ounces Neufchâtel cheese, softened
⅓ cup peach preserves
1 cup (4 ounces) shredded fat-free Cheddar cheese
½ cup packed stemmed and washed fresh spinach leaves
3 ounces thinly sliced regular or smoked turkey breast

1. Spread each tortilla evenly with 1 ounce Neufchâtel cheese; cover with thin layer of preserves. Sprinkle with ¼ cup Cheddar cheese.

2. Arrange spinach leaves and turkey over Cheddar cheese. Roll up tortillas; trim ends. Cover and refrigerate until ready to serve.

3. Cut "rollers" crosswise in half or diagonally into 1-inch pieces.

Makes 4 servings

oven-fried tex-mex onion rings

roasted eggplant rolls

nutrients per serving:

2 rolls with
2 tablespoons
spaghetti sauce

Calories: 77
Carbohydrate: 12 g
Dietary Fiber: <1 g
Total Fat: 3 g
Calories From Fat: 27%
Saturated Fat: <1 g
Cholesterol: 0 mg
Sodium: 213 mg
Protein: 3 g

Exchanges: 2 Vegetable, ½ Fat

  2 **medium eggplants (¾ pound each)**
  2 **tablespoons lemon juice**
  1 **teaspoon olive oil**
  4 **tablespoons (2 ounces) fat-free cream cheese**
  2 **tablespoons fat-free sour cream**
  1 **green onion, minced**
  4 **sun-dried tomatoes (packed in oil), rinsed, drained and minced**
  1 **clove garlic, minced**
  ¼ **teaspoon dried oregano leaves**
  ⅛ **teaspoon black pepper**
 16 **fresh spinach leaves, washed, stemmed and dried**
  1 **cup bottled prepared spaghetti sauce**

1. Preheat oven to 450°F. Spray 2 nonstick baking sheets with nonstick cooking spray; set aside.

2. Trim ends from eggplants; cut eggplants lengthwise into ¼-inch-thick slices. Discard outside slices that are mostly skin. (You will have about 16 slices total.)

3. Combine lemon juice and olive oil in small bowl; brush lightly over both sides of eggplant slices. Arrange slices in single layer on baking sheets. Bake 22 to 24 minutes or until slightly golden brown, turning once. Transfer slices to plate; cool.

4. Meanwhile, stir together cream cheese, sour cream, green onion, tomatoes, garlic, oregano and pepper in small bowl until blended.

5. Spread about 1 teaspoon cream cheese mixture evenly over each eggplant slice. Arrange spinach leaf on top, leaving ½-inch border. Roll up, beginning at small end; lay rolls, seam sides down, on serving platter. (If making ahead, cover and refrigerate up to 2 days. Bring to room temperature before serving.) Serve with warmed spaghetti sauce.   *Makes 8 servings (2 rolls each)*

roasted eggplant rolls

smoked salmon appetizers

¼ cup reduced-fat or fat-free cream cheese, softened
1 tablespoon chopped fresh dill *or* 1 teaspoon dried dill weed
⅛ teaspoon ground red pepper
4 ounces thinly sliced smoked salmon or lox
24 melba toast rounds or other low-fat crackers
Fresh dill sprigs, for garnish (optional)

1. Combine cream cheese, dill and red pepper in small bowl; stir to blend. Spread evenly over each slice of salmon. Roll up salmon slices jelly-roll fashion. Place on plate; cover with plastic wrap. Chill at least 1 hour or up to 4 hours before serving.

2. Using sharp knife, cut salmon rolls crosswise into ¾-inch pieces. Place pieces, cut side down, on melba rounds. Garnish each salmon roll with dill sprig, if desired. Serve cold or at room temperature. *Makes about 2 dozen appetizers*

nutrients per serving:

1 smoked salmon appetizer
Calories: 80
Carbohydrate: 10 g
Dietary Fiber: 1 g
Total Fat: 2 g
Calories From Fat: 21%
Saturated Fat: 1 g
Cholesterol: 6 mg
Sodium: 241 mg
Protein: 6 g
Exchanges: ½ Starch, ½ Lean Meat

super nachos

12 large baked low-fat tortilla chips (about 1½ ounces)
½ cup (2 ounces) shredded reduced-fat Cheddar cheese
¼ cup fat-free refried beans
2 tablespoons chunky salsa

Microwave Directions

1. Arrange chips in single layer on large microwavable plate. Sprinkle cheese evenly over chips. Spoon 1 teaspoon beans over each chip; top with ½ teaspoon salsa.

2. Microwave at MEDIUM (50% power) 1½ minutes; rotate dish. Microwave 1 to 1½ minutes more or until cheese is melted. *Makes 2 servings*

Conventional Directions: Substitute foil-covered baking sheet for microwavable plate. Assemble nachos as directed on prepared baking sheet. Bake at 350°F 10 to 12 minutes or until cheese is melted.

nutrients per serving:

6 nachos
Calories: 176
Carbohydrate: 23 g
Dietary Fiber: 2 g
Total Fat: 5 g
Calories From Fat: 26%
Saturated Fat: 2 g
Cholesterol: 16 mg
Sodium: 683 mg
Protein: 10 g
Exchanges: 1½ Starch, 1 Lean Meat

smoked salmon appetizers

spicy vegetable quesadillas

nutrients per serving:

1 quesadilla
(3 wedges)
Calories: 153
Carbohydrate: 23 g
Dietary Fiber: 1 g
Total Fat: 4 g
Calories From Fat: 22%
Saturated Fat: 1 g
Cholesterol: 8 mg
Sodium: 201 mg
Protein: 7 g
Exchanges: 1½ Starch,
½ Vegetable, ½ Lean Meat

Nonstick cooking spray
1 small zucchini, chopped
½ cup *each* chopped onion and chopped green bell pepper
2 cloves garlic, minced
½ teaspoon *each* chili powder and ground cumin
8 (6-inch) flour tortillas
1 cup (4 ounces) shredded reduced-fat Cheddar cheese
¼ cup chopped fresh cilantro

1. Spray large nonstick skillet with cooking spray. Heat over medium heat until hot. Add zucchini, onion, bell pepper, garlic, chili powder and cumin; cook and stir 3 to 4 minutes or until vegetables are crisp-tender. Remove vegetables; set aside. Wipe skillet clean.

2. Spoon vegetable mixture evenly over half of each tortilla. Sprinkle each evenly with cheese and cilantro. Fold each tortilla in half.

3. Spray same skillet with cooking spray. Add tortillas; heat 1 to 2 minutes per side over medium heat or until lightly browned. Cut into thirds before serving.

Makes 8 servings

avocado salsa

nutrients per serving:

2 tablespoons salsa
Calories: 13
Carbohydrate: 1 g
Dietary Fiber: <1 g
Total Fat: 1 g
Calories From Fat: 60%
Saturated Fat: <1 g
Cholesterol: 0 mg
Sodium: 38 mg
Protein: <1 g
Exchanges: Free

1 medium avocado, peeled and diced
1 cup chopped seeded peeled cucumber
1 cup chopped onion
1 Anaheim chili, seeded and chopped*
½ cup chopped fresh tomato
2 tablespoons chopped fresh cilantro
½ teaspoon salt
¼ teaspoon hot pepper sauce

*Chili peppers can sting and irritate the skin. Wear rubber gloves when handling peppers and do not touch eyes. Wash hands after handling chili peppers.

Combine avocado, cucumber, onion, chili, tomato, cilantro, salt and hot pepper sauce in medium bowl; mix well. Refrigerate, covered, at least 1 hour to allow flavors to blend. Serve as dip or condiment.

Makes about 32 servings (4 cups)

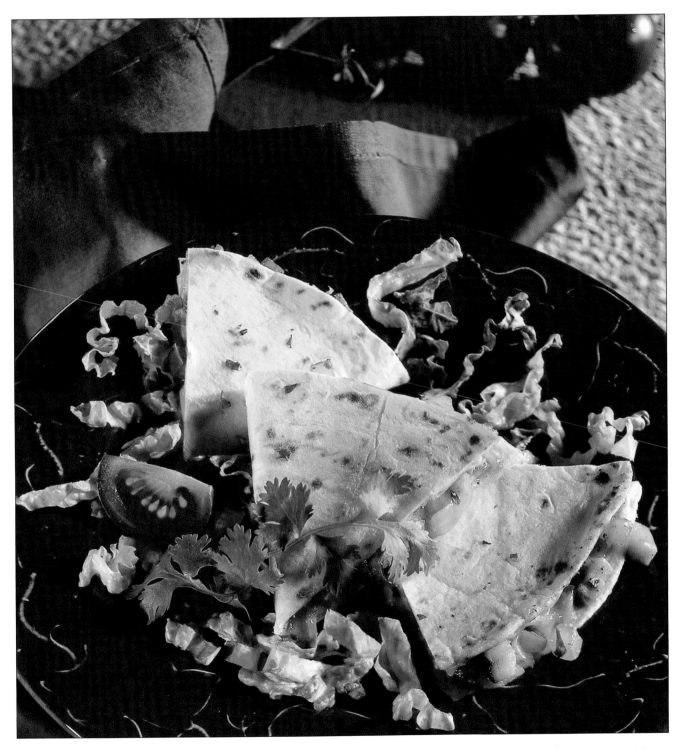

spicy vegetable quesadillas

bruschetta

nutrients per serving:

1 bruschetta slice

Calories: 90
Carbohydrate: 17 g
Dietary Fiber: <1 g
Total Fat: 2 g
Calories From Fat: 20%
Saturated Fat: <1 g
Cholesterol: 0 mg
Sodium: 194 mg
Protein: 3 g

Exchanges: 1 Starch,
½ Lean Meat

   Nonstick cooking spray
 1 cup thinly sliced onion
 ½ cup chopped seeded tomato
 2 tablespoons capers
 ¼ teaspoon black pepper
 3 cloves garlic, finely chopped
 1 teaspoon olive oil
 4 slices French bread
 ½ cup (2 ounces) shredded reduced-fat Monterey Jack cheese

1. Spray large nonstick skillet with cooking spray. Heat over medium heat until hot. Add onion; cook and stir 5 minutes. Stir in tomato, capers and pepper. Cook 3 minutes.

2. Preheat broiler. Combine garlic and olive oil in small bowl. Brush bread slices with mixture. Top with onion mixture; sprinkle with cheese. Place on baking sheet. Broil 3 minutes or until cheese melts.
Makes 4 servings

mexican bean dip

nutrients per serving:

2 tablespoons dip

Calories: 56
Carbohydrate: 9 g
Fiber: 3 g
Total Fat: 2 g
Calories From Fat: 32%
Saturated Fat: <1 g
Cholesterol: 0 mg
Sodium: 3 mg
Protein: 3 g

Exchanges: ½ Starch,
½ Vegetable

 1 can (15 ounces) red kidney beans, rinsed and drained
 1 medium avocado, chopped
 2 tablespoons lemon juice
 2 tablespoons tomato paste
 1 red chili, finely chopped (optional)
 2 cloves garlic, minced
 1 tablespoon EQUAL® SPOONFUL*
 1 green onion, sliced
 ¼ cup parsley, chopped

*May substitute 1½ packets Equal® sweetener.

● Process kidney beans, avocado, lemon juice, tomato paste, chili, garlic and Equal® Spoonful in food processor until well blended. Stir in green onion and 3 tablespoons parsley. Sprinkle with remaining parsley.
Makes 1¾ cups

bruschetta

light lunches

mandarin turkey salad with buttermilk-herb dressing

Buttermilk-Herb Dressing (recipe follows)
1 can (about 14 ounces) fat-free reduced-sodium chicken broth
1¼ pounds turkey tenderloins, cut in half lengthwise
½ teaspoon dried basil leaves
½ pound (about 8 cups) mesclun salad greens, washed and dried
2 pounds (about 10 cups) raw cut-up vegetables such as broccoli florets, red or yellow bell peppers, carrots and red onion
1 can (11 ounces) mandarin orange segments, drained

1. Prepare Buttermilk-Herb Dressing; set aside.

2. Place broth in medium saucepan; bring to a boil over high heat. Add turkey and basil. Return to a boil; reduce heat. Simmer, covered, 12 to 14 minutes or until turkey is no longer pink.

3. Remove turkey from broth. When cool enough to handle, shred turkey into strips.

4. Arrange salad greens on individual plates. Divide turkey evenly over salad greens. Arrange vegetables and orange segments around turkey. Drizzle each serving with 2 tablespoons Buttermilk-Herb Dressing. *Makes 6 servings*

buttermilk-herb dressing

½ cup plus 1 tablespoon nonfat buttermilk
3 tablespoons raspberry-flavored vinegar
1 tablespoon chopped fresh basil leaves
1½ teaspoons snipped fresh chives
¼ teaspoon minced garlic

Place all ingredients in small bowl; stir to combine. Store, covered, in refrigerator up to 2 days. *Makes about ¾ cup*

mandarin turkey salad with buttermilk-herb dressing

tangy italian chicken sandwiches

**2 cups (8 ounces) chopped cooked boneless skinless chicken or
  turkey breast**
⅓ cup drained bottled hot or mild pickled vegetables (jardinière)
2 ounces reduced-fat provolone cheese slices, diced
¼ cup chopped fresh parsley
3 tablespoons prepared reduced-fat Italian salad dressing
¼ teaspoon dried oregano leaves
4 pita bread rounds (2 ounces each)
8 leaves romaine or red leaf lettuce

1. Combine chicken, pickled vegetables, cheese, parsley, dressing and oregano in medium bowl; mix well.

2. Cut pitas in half crosswise; gently open. Line each half with lettuce leaf. Divide chicken mixture evenly among pita pockets. *Makes 4 servings*

nutrients per serving:

2 filled pita halves
Calories: 330
Carbohydrate: 39 g
Dietary Fiber: 6 g
Total Fat: 7 g
Calories From Fat: 20%
Saturated Fat: 3 g
Cholesterol: 53 mg
Sodium: 610 mg
Protein: 28 g

Exchanges: 2½ Starch, 2 Lean Meat, ½ Fat

garden tuna salad

1 can (6 ounces) tuna packed in water, drained
1 medium carrot, chopped
1 rib celery, chopped
½ cup reduced-fat Monterey Jack cheese cubes (¼ inch each)
¼ cup frozen green peas, thawed and drained
¼ teaspoon dried parsley flakes
⅓ cup prepared reduced-fat Italian salad dressing
2 pita bread rounds (2 ounces each)
4 lettuce leaves
4 tomato slices

1. Place tuna in large bowl; break into chunks. Add carrot, celery, cheese, peas and parsley; toss to blend. Pour dressing over tuna mixture; toss lightly to coat.

2. Cut each pita in half crosswise; gently open. Place lettuce leaf and tomato slice in each pita half. Divide tuna salad evenly among pita pockets. *Makes 4 servings*

nutrients per serving:

1 pita half with about ½ cup tuna salad, 1 lettuce leaf and 1 tomato slice
Calories: 213
Carbohydrate: 22 g
Dietary Fiber: 4 g
Total Fat: 6 g
Calories From Fat: 23%
Saturated Fat: 2 g
Cholesterol: 24 mg
Sodium: 605 mg
Protein: 19 g

Exchanges: 1½ Starch, 2 Lean Meat

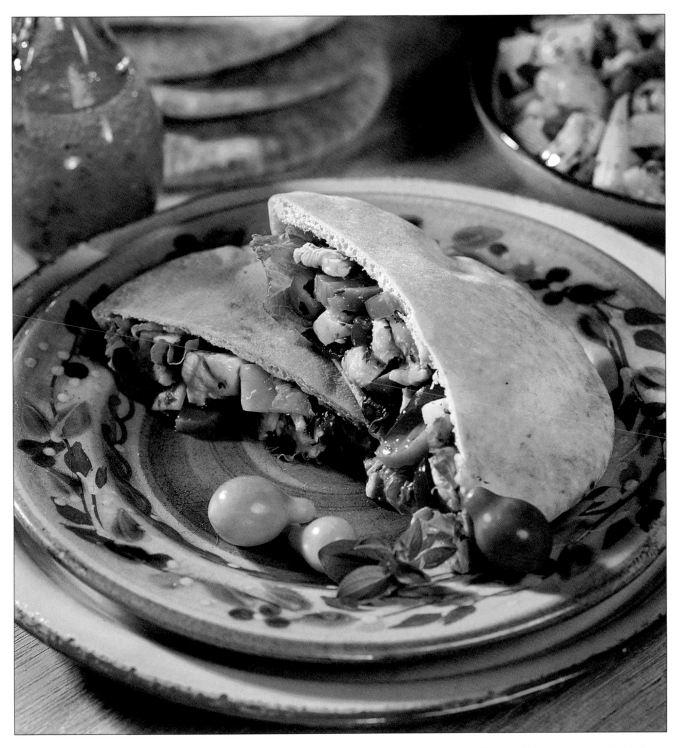

tangy italian chicken sandwiches

mexican pita pile-ups

4 whole-grain pita bread rounds
1 cup cooked, diced, boneless skinless chicken breast
1 tablespoon lime juice
1 teaspoon ground cumin
¼ cup chopped mild green chilies*
1 cup chopped seeded tomato
¼ cup chopped fresh cilantro leaves
1 can (2¼ ounces) sliced ripe olives, drained
1 cup shredded reduced-fat sharp cheddar cheese

Chili peppers can sting and irritate the skin. Wear rubber gloves when handling chilies and do not touch eyes. Wash hands after handling chilies.

Microwave Directions

1. Place pita rounds on work surface. Top each with ¼ cup chicken, lime juice, cumin, chilies, tomato, cilantro, olives and cheese. Place each uncooked pile-up in quart-size resealable plastic food storage bag; seal. Refrigerate until ready to serve.

2. To serve, place pita on microwavable plate. Microwave at HIGH 1 minute or until cheese is melted. Let stand 2 to 3 minutes or until crust is slightly firm.

Makes 4 servings

nutrients per serving:

1 pile-up
Calories: 287
Carbohydrate: 33 g
Dietary Fiber: 7 g
Total Fat: 9 g
Calories From Fat: 25%
Saturated Fat: 4 g
Cholesterol: 37 mg
Sodium: 731 mg
Protein: 26 g
Exchanges: 2 Starch, 3 Lean Meat

huevos ranchwich

¼ cup EGG BEATERS®
1 teaspoon diced green chiles
1 whole wheat hamburger roll, split and toasted
1 tablespoon thick and chunky salsa, heated
1 tablespoon shredded reduced-fat Cheddar and Monterey Jack cheese blend

On lightly greased griddle or skillet, pour Egg Beaters® into lightly greased 4-inch egg ring or biscuit cutter. Sprinkle with chiles. Cook 2 to 3 minutes or until bottom of egg patty is set. Remove egg ring and turn egg patty over. Cook 1 to 2 minutes longer or until done.

To serve, place egg patty on bottom of roll. Top with salsa, cheese and roll top.

Makes 1 sandwich

nutrients per serving:

1 sandwich
Calories: 168
Carbohydrate: 21 g
Dietary Fiber: 2 g
Total Fat: 4 g
Calories From Fat: 20%
Saturated Fat: 1 g
Cholesterol: 5 mg
Sodium: 495 mg
Protein: 13 g
Exchanges: 1½ Starch, 1 Lean Meat

mexican pita pile-up

turkey vegetable chili mac

Nonstick cooking spray
¾ pound 93% lean ground turkey
½ cup chopped onion
2 cloves garlic, minced
1 can (about 15 ounces) black beans, rinsed and drained
1 can (14½ ounces) Mexican-style stewed tomatoes, undrained
1 can (14½ ounces) no-salt-added diced tomatoes, undrained
1 cup frozen corn
1 teaspoon Mexican seasoning
½ cup uncooked elbow macaroni
⅓ cup reduced-fat sour cream

1. Spray large nonstick saucepan or Dutch oven with cooking spray; heat over medium heat until hot. Add turkey, onion and garlic; cook and stir 5 minutes or until turkey is no longer pink.

2. Stir beans, tomatoes with juice, corn and Mexican seasoning into saucepan; bring to a boil over high heat. Cover; reduce heat to low. Simmer 15 minutes, stirring occasionally.

3. Meanwhile, cook pasta according to package directions, omitting salt. Rinse and drain pasta; stir into saucepan. Simmer, uncovered, 2 to 3 minutes or until heated through.

4. Top each serving with dollop of sour cream. Garnish as desired.

Makes 6 servings

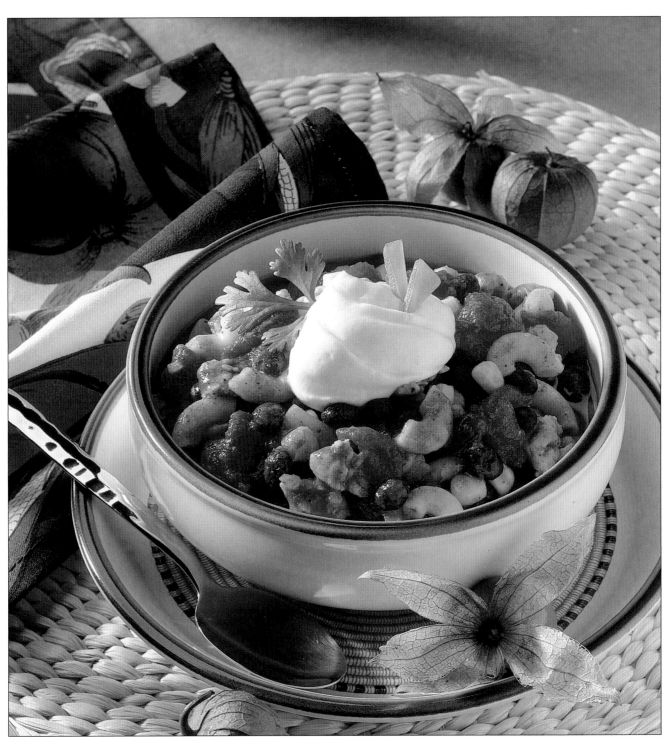

turkey vegetable chili mac

raspberry mango salad

nutrients per serving:

¼ of total recipe

Calories: 98
Carbohydrate: 12 g
Dietary Fiber: 2 g
Total Fat: 8 g
Calories From Fat: 74%
Saturated Fat: 3 g
Cholesterol: 8 mg
Sodium: 227 mg
Protein: 3 g

Exchanges: ½ Vegetable, 2 Fat

2 cups arugula
1 cup torn Bibb or Boston lettuce
1 cup diced mango
¾ cup fresh raspberries
½ cup watercress, stems removed
¼ cup (1½ ounces) crumbled blue cheese
1 tablespoon olive oil
1 tablespoon water
1 tablespoon raspberry vinegar
⅛ teaspoon salt
⅛ teaspoon black pepper

1. Combine arugula, lettuce, mango, raspberries, watercress and cheese in medium bowl.

2. Place remaining ingredients in small jar; shake to combine. Pour over salad; toss to coat. Serve immediately.

Makes 4 servings

vegetable-chicken noodle soup

nutrients per serving:

about 1 cup soup

Calories: 98
Carbohydrate: 12 g
Dietary Fiber: 1 g
Total Fat: 2 g
Calories From Fat: 14%
Saturated Fat: <1 g
Cholesterol: 18 mg
Sodium: 73 mg
Protein: 10 g

Exchanges: ½ Starch, ½ Vegetable, 1 Lean Meat

¼ cup chopped celery
¼ cup thinly sliced leek (white part only)
¼ cup chopped carrot
¼ cup chopped turnip
3 cups fat-free reduced-sodium chicken broth, divided
1 teaspoon minced fresh parsley
½ teaspoon fresh thyme *or* pinch dried thyme leaves
½ teaspoon fresh rosemary *or* pinch dried rosemary leaves, crushed
½ teaspoon balsamic vinegar
⅛ teaspoon black pepper
½ ounce uncooked yolk-free wide noodles
¼ cup diced cooked boneless skinless chicken breast

1. Place celery, leek, carrot, turnip and ⅓ cup broth in medium saucepan. Cover; cook over medium heat 12 to 15 minutes or until vegetables are tender, stirring occasionally.

2. Stir in remaining broth, parsley, thyme, rosemary, vinegar and pepper; bring to a boil. Add noodles; cook until noodles are tender. Stir in chicken. Reduce heat to medium; simmer until heated through.

Makes 2 servings

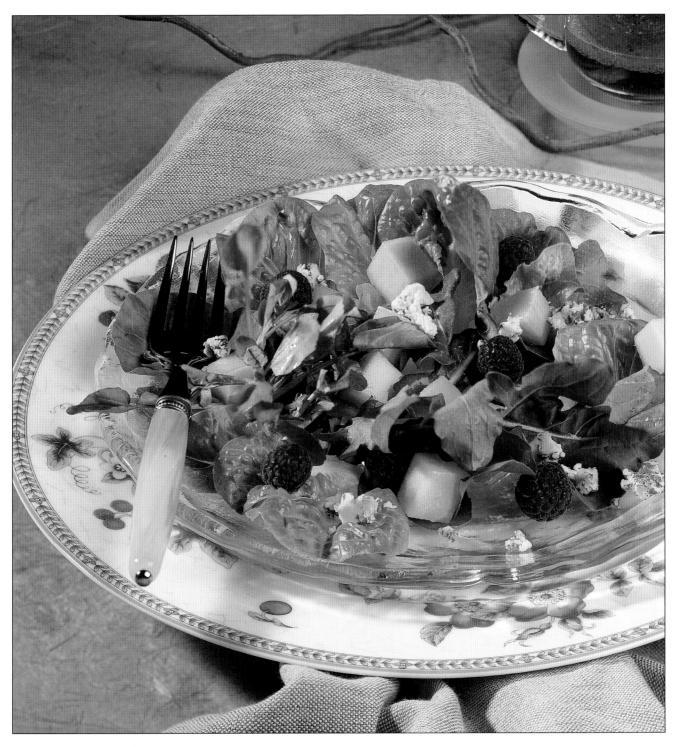

raspberry mango salad

tuscan chicken with white beans

nutrients per serving:
1½ cups soup
Calories: 215
Carbohydrate: 24 g
Dietary Fiber: 7 g
Total Fat: 6 g
Calories From Fat: 25%
Saturated Fat: 2 g
Cholesterol: 34 mg
Sodium: 321 mg
Protein: 17 g

Exchanges: 1 Starch, 1½ Vegetable, 2 Lean Meat

- 1 large fresh fennel bulb (about ¾ pound)
- 1 teaspoon olive oil
- 8 ounces boneless skinless chicken thighs, cut into ¾-inch pieces
- 1 teaspoon dried rosemary leaves, crushed
- ½ teaspoon black pepper
- 1 can (14½ ounces) no-salt-added stewed tomatoes, undrained
- 1 can (about 14 ounces) fat-free reduced-sodium chicken broth
- 1 can (about 15 ounces) cannellini beans, rinsed and drained
- Hot pepper sauce (optional)

1. Cut off and reserve ¼ cup chopped feathery fennel tops. Chop bulb into ½-inch pieces. Heat oil in large saucepan over medium heat. Add chopped fennel bulb; cook 5 minutes, stirring occasionally.

2. Sprinkle chicken with rosemary and pepper; add to saucepan. Cook and stir 2 minutes. Add tomatoes with juice and chicken broth; bring to a boil. Cover; simmer 10 minutes. Stir in beans; simmer, uncovered, 15 minutes or until chicken is cooked through and sauce thickens. Season to taste with hot sauce, if desired. Ladle into 4 shallow bowls; top with reserved fennel tops. *Makes 4 servings*

chunky chicken stew

nutrients per serving:
1 bowl stew (½ of total recipe)
Calories: 287
Carbohydrate: 31 g
Dietary Fiber: 8 g
Total Fat: 6 g
Calories From Fat: 18%
Saturated Fat: 1 g
Cholesterol: 66 mg
Sodium: 337 mg
Protein: 30 g

Exchanges: 6 Vegetable, 3 Lean Meat

- 1 teaspoon olive oil
- 1 small onion, chopped
- 1 cup thinly sliced carrots
- 1 cup fat-free reduced-sodium chicken broth
- 1 can (14½ ounces) no-salt-added diced tomatoes, undrained
- 1 cup diced cooked chicken breast
- 3 cups sliced kale or baby spinach leaves

1. Heat oil in large saucepan over medium-high heat. Add onion; cook and stir about 5 minutes or until golden brown. Stir in carrots, then broth; bring to a boil.

2. Reduce heat; simmer, uncovered, 5 minutes. Add tomatoes with juice; simmer 5 minutes or until carrots are tender. Add chicken; heat through. Add kale, stirring until kale is wilted. Simmer 1 minute. Ladle into 2 soup bowls. *Makes 2 servings*

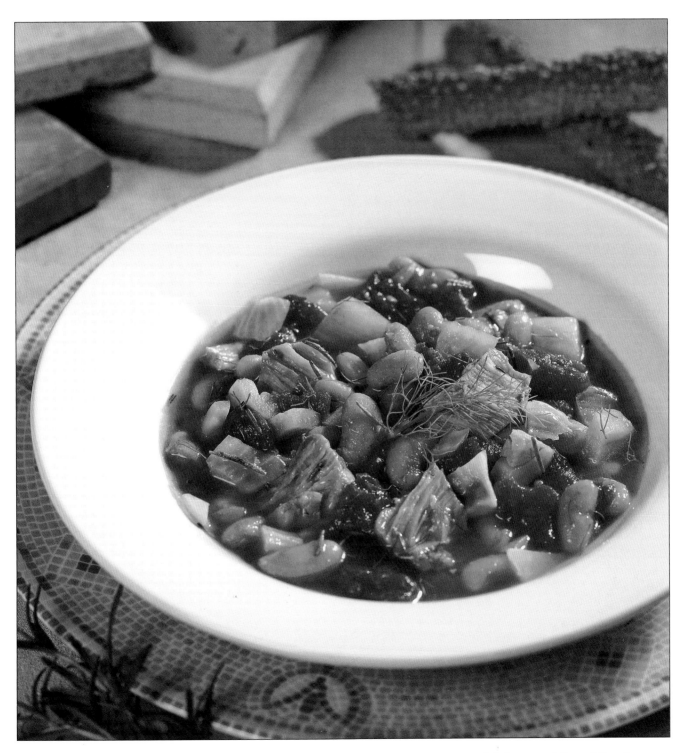

tuscan chicken with white beans

pasta and tuna filled peppers

nutrients per serving:

1 filled pepper (without cheese topping)
Calories: 216
Carbohydrate: 27 g
Dietary Fiber: 2 g
Total Fat: 4 g
Calories From Fat: 16%
Saturated Fat: 1 g
Cholesterol: 26 mg
Sodium: 574 mg
Protein: 19 g

Exchanges: 1 Starch, 2 Vegetable, 2 Lean Meat

¾ cup uncooked ditalini pasta
4 large green bell peppers
1 cup chopped seeded fresh tomatoes
1 can (6 ounces) white tuna packed in water, drained and flaked
½ cup chopped celery
½ cup (2 ounces) shredded reduced-fat Cheddar cheese
¼ cup fat-free mayonnaise or salad dressing
1 teaspoon salt-free garlic and herb seasoning
2 tablespoons shredded reduced-fat Cheddar cheese (optional)

Microwave Directions

1. Cook pasta according to package directions, omitting salt. Rinse and drain. Set aside.

2. Cut thin slice from top of each pepper. Remove seeds and membranes from insides of peppers. Rinse peppers; place, cut side down, on paper towels to drain.*

3. Combine cooked pasta, tomatoes, tuna, celery, ½ cup cheese, mayonnaise and seasoning in large bowl until well blended; spoon evenly into pepper shells.

4. Place peppers on large microwavable plate; cover with waxed paper. Microwave at HIGH 7 to 8 minutes, turning halfway through cooking time. Top evenly with remaining 2 tablespoons cheese before serving, if desired. Garnish as desired.

Makes 4 servings

For more tender peppers, cook in boiling water 2 minutes. Rinse with cold water; drain upside down on paper towels before filling.

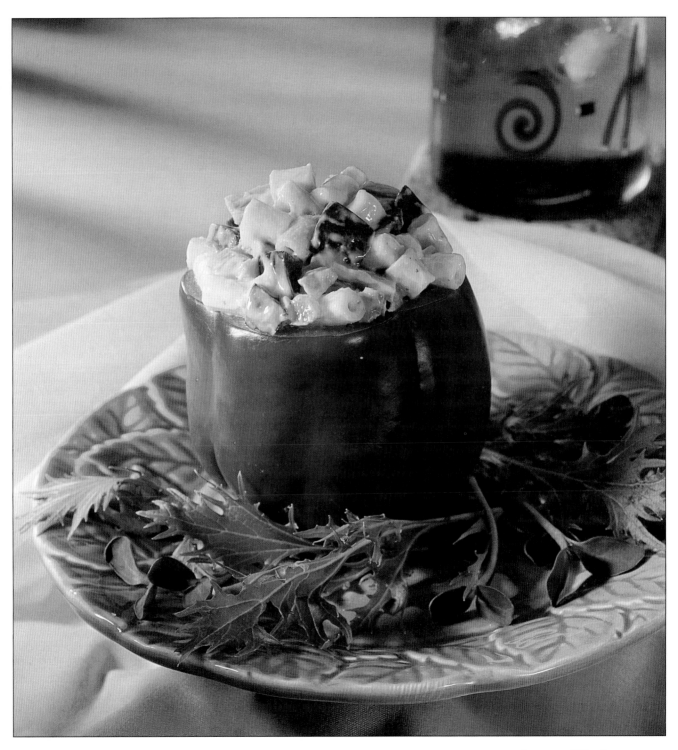

pasta and tuna filled pepper

nutrients per serving:

1 sandwich
Calories: 282
Carbohydrate: 37 g
Dietary Fiber: 7 g
Total Fat: 7 g
Calories From Fat: 19%
Saturated Fat: 1 g
Cholesterol: 47 mg
Sodium: 282 mg
Protein: 27 g
Exchanges: 2 Starch,
1½ Vegetable,
2 Lean Meat

turkey sandwiches with roasted bell peppers

2 large red bell peppers
8 slices whole-grain or millet bread
¼ cup reduced-fat mayonnaise
4 romaine lettuce leaves *or* 8 spinach leaves
8 thin slices red onion
8 ounces thinly sliced skinless roasted turkey breast
8 large basil leaves (optional)

1. Preheat broiler. Cut bell peppers into quarters; discard stems, membranes and seeds. Place peppers, skin side up, on foil-lined baking sheet. Broil 3 inches from heat 10 minutes or until skin is blackened. Wrap peppers in foil from baking sheet; let stand 10 minutes. Peel off and discard skin.

2. Spread 4 bread slices with mayonnaise. Top with lettuce, onion, turkey, peppers and basil, if desired. Top with remaining 4 bread slices. *Makes 4 servings*

tip

Cool and Creamy Pea Salad with Cucumbers and Red Onion (page 258) makes a great side dish for this healthy, tasty sandwich.

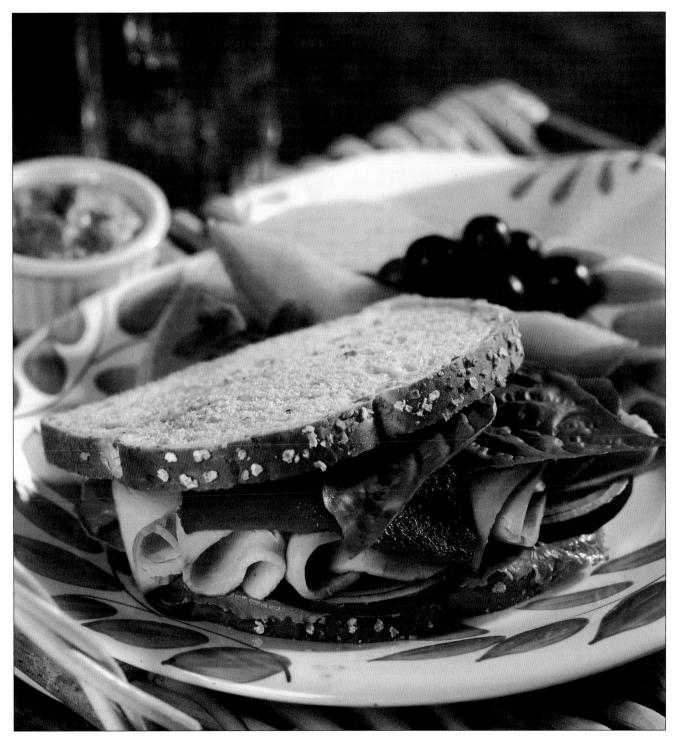

turkey sandwich with roasted bell peppers

shrimp étouffée

nutrients per serving:

1 bowl étouffée with ½ cup rice

Calories: 306
Carbohydrate: 32 g
Dietary Fiber: 1 g
Total Fat: 7 g
Calories From Fat: 20%
Saturated Fat: 1 g
Cholesterol: 219 mg
Sodium: 454 mg
Protein: 27 g

Exchanges: 1½ Starch, 1½ Vegetable, 3 Lean Meat

3 tablespoons canola oil
¼ cup all-purpose flour
1 cup chopped onion
1 cup chopped green bell pepper
½ cup chopped carrot
½ cup chopped celery
4 cloves garlic, minced
1 can (14½ ounces) clear vegetable broth
1 bottle (8 ounces) clam juice
½ teaspoon salt
2½ pounds uncooked large shrimp, peeled and deveined
1 teaspoon red pepper flakes
1 teaspoon hot pepper sauce
4 cups hot cooked white or basmati rice
½ cup chopped flat leaf parsley
    Additional hot pepper sauce (optional)

1. Heat oil in Dutch oven over medium heat. Add flour; cook and stir 10 to 15 minutes or until flour mixture is deep golden brown. Add onion, bell pepper, carrot, celery and garlic; cook and stir 5 minutes.

2. Stir in broth, clam juice and salt; bring to a boil. Simmer, uncovered, 10 minutes or until vegetables are tender. Stir in shrimp, red pepper flakes and hot pepper sauce; simmer 6 to 8 minutes or until shrimp are opaque.

3. Ladle into 8 shallow bowls; top each with ½ cup rice. Sprinkle with parsley. Serve with additional pepper sauce, if desired.   *Makes 8 servings*

shrimp étouffée

grilled mozzarella & roasted red pepper sandwich

nutrients per serving:

1 sandwich
(2 sandwich halves)
Calories: 303
Carbohydrate: 35 g
Dietary Fiber: 2 g
Total Fat: 9 g
Calories From Fat: 29%
Saturated Fat: 5 g
Cholesterol: 25 mg
Sodium: 727 mg
Protein: 16 g

Exchanges: 2 Starch, 1 Vegetable, 1 Lean Meat, 1½ Fat

1 tablespoon reduced-fat olive oil vinaigrette or prepared reduced-fat Italian salad dressing
2 slices (2 ounces) Italian-style sandwich bread
 Basil leaves (optional)
⅓ cup roasted red peppers, rinsed, drained and patted dry
2 slices (1 ounce each) part-skim mozzarella or reduced-fat Swiss cheese
 Nonstick olive oil cooking spray

1. Brush dressing onto one side of one slice of bread; top with basil, if desired, peppers, cheese and second bread slice. Lightly spray both sides of sandwich with cooking spray.

2. Heat skillet over medium heat until hot. Place sandwich in skillet; grill 4 to 5 minutes on each side or until brown and cheese is melted. Cut in half before serving, if desired.

Makes 1 sandwich

sunburst chicken salad

nutrients per serving:

½ of total recipe
Calories: 195
Carbohydrate: 18 g
Dietary Fiber: 2 g
Total Fat: 6 g
Calories From Fat: 29%
Saturated Fat: 1 g
Cholesterol: 39 mg
Sodium: 431 mg
Protein: 18 g

Exchanges: 1 Fruit, 2 Lean Meat, ½ Fat

1 tablespoon fat-free mayonnaise
1 tablespoon fat-free sour cream
2 teaspoons frozen orange juice concentrate, thawed
¼ teaspoon grated fresh orange peel
1 boneless skinless chicken breast, cooked and chopped
1 large kiwi, thinly sliced
⅓ cup canned mandarin oranges, drained
¼ cup finely chopped celery
4 lettuce leaves, washed
2 tablespoons coarsely chopped cashews

Combine mayonnaise, sour cream, orange juice concentrate and orange peel in small bowl. Add chicken, kiwi, oranges and celery; toss to coat. Cover; refrigerate 2 hours. Serve on lettuce leaves. Top with cashews.

Makes 2 servings

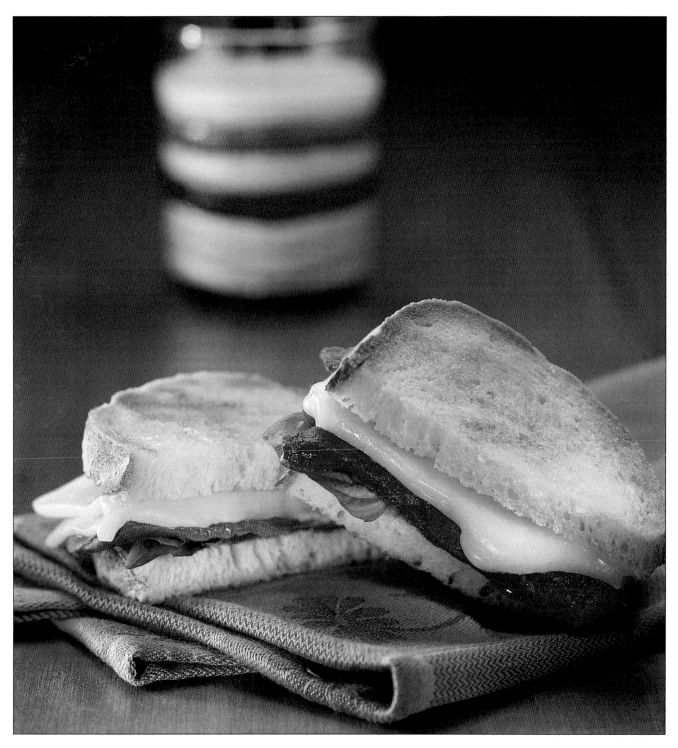

grilled mozzarella & roasted red pepper sandwich

chicken and spinach salad

nutrients per serving:

¼ of total recipe
Calories: 218
Carbohydrate: 23 g
Dietary Fiber: 3 g
Total Fat: 4 g
Calories From Fat: 15%
Saturated Fat: 1 g
Cholesterol: 55 mg
Sodium: 361 mg
Protein: 23 g

Exchanges: 1 Fruit,
1½ Vegetable,
2 Lean Meat

¾ pound chicken tenders
Nonstick cooking spray
4 cups washed, stemmed and shredded spinach
2 cups washed and torn romaine lettuce
8 thin slices red onion
2 tablespoons (½ ounce) crumbled blue cheese
1 large grapefruit, peeled and sectioned
½ cup frozen citrus blend concentrate, thawed
¼ cup prepared fat-free Italian salad dressing

1. Cut chicken into 2×½-inch strips. Spray large nonstick skillet with cooking spray; heat over medium heat until hot. Add chicken; cook and stir 5 minutes or until no longer pink in center. Remove from skillet; set aside.

2. Divide spinach, lettuce, onion, cheese, grapefruit and chicken among 4 salad plates. Combine citrus blend concentrate and Italian dressing in small bowl; drizzle over salads. Garnish with assorted greens, if desired.   *Makes 4 servings*

grilled portobello open-faced sandwich

nutrients per serving:

1 sandwich
Calories: 155
Carbohydrate: 17 g
Dietary Fiber: 1 g
Total Fat: 8 g
Calories From Fat: 44%
Saturated Fat: 1 g
Cholesterol: 2 mg
Sodium: 300 mg
Protein: 4 g

Exchanges: 1 Starch,
1 Vegetable, 1½ Fat

1 portobello mushroom cap, rinsed and stem removed
2 teaspoons balsamic vinegar
1 tablespoon prepared pesto sauce
1 slice bread, toasted
1 teaspoon grated Parmesan cheese

1. Preheat broiler. Sprinkle mushroom cap with balsamic vinegar. Place on rack under broiler about 4 inches from heat. Cook 3 to 4 minutes on each side or until tender.

2. Spread pesto onto toast. Top with mushroom cap and sprinkle with Parmesan cheese. Serve immediately.   *Makes 1 serving*

chicken and spinach salad

nutrients per serving:

1 turnover
Calories: 188
Carbohydrate: 24 g
Dietary Fiber: 3 g
Total Fat: 6 g
Calories From Fat: 28%
Saturated Fat: 2 g
Cholesterol: 17 mg
Sodium: 502 mg
Protein: 10 g

Exchanges: 1½ Starch,
½ Vegetable,
½ Lean Meat, ½ Fat

pizza turnovers

5 ounces reduced-fat mild Italian bulk turkey sausage
½ cup prepared pizza sauce
1 package (10 ounces) refrigerated pizza dough
⅓ cup shredded reduced-fat Italian cheese blend

1. Preheat oven to 425°F. Cook and stir sausage in nonstick saucepan over medium-high heat until browned. Drain fat. Add pizza sauce. Cook and stir until hot.

2. Spray baking sheet with nonstick olive oil cooking spray. Unroll pizza dough onto baking sheet. Pat into 12×8-inch rectangle. Cut into 6 (4×4-inch) squares. Divide sausage mixture evenly among squares. Sprinkle with cheese. Lift 1 corner of each square; fold over filling to opposite corner. Press edges with tines of fork to seal.

3. Bake 11 to 13 minutes or until golden brown. Serve immediately or follow directions for freezing and reheating. *Makes 6 servings*

Note: To freeze turnovers, remove to wire rack to cool 30 minutes. Individually wrap in plastic wrap, or place in freezer container or plastic freezer bag and freeze. To reheat, preheat oven to 400°F. Unwrap turnovers. Place in ungreased baking pan. Cover loosely with foil. Bake 18 to 22 minutes or until hot. Or, place one turnover on a paper-towel-lined microwavable plate. Heat on DEFROST (30% power) 3 to 3½ minutes or until hot, turning once.

nutrients per serving:

½ of total recipe
Calories: 262
Carbohydrate: 26 g
Dietary Fiber: 2 g
Total Fat: 9 g
Calories From Fat: 32%
Saturated Fat: 2 g
Cholesterol: 21 mg
Sodium: 627 mg
Protein: 18 g

Exchanges: 1½ Starch,
1 Vegetable, 2 Lean Meat,
½ Fat

salmon pasta salad

1 cup cooked medium pasta shells
1 can (6 ounces) canned red salmon, rinsed and drained
½ cup finely chopped celery
2 tablespoons finely chopped red bell pepper
2 tablespoons chopped fresh parsley
2 tablespoons fat-free mayonnaise
1 green onion, finely chopped
1 tablespoon lemon juice
2 teaspoons capers
⅛ teaspoon paprika

Combine all ingredients in medium bowl. Cover; refrigerate before serving.
Makes 2 servings

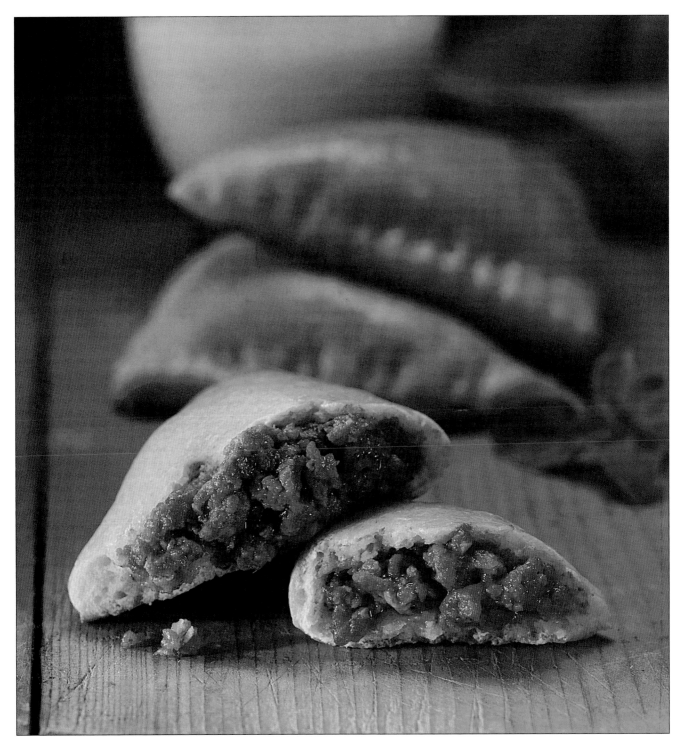

pizza turnovers

broiled turkey burgers

   1 pound 93% lean ground turkey
   ¼ cup finely chopped green onions
   ¼ cup finely chopped fresh parsley
   2 tablespoons dry red wine
   1 teaspoon dried Italian seasoning
   ¼ teaspoon salt
   ¼ teaspoon black pepper
   4 whole wheat hamburger buns
      Toppings: lettuce, grilled pineapple slices and bell pepper strips
      (optional)

1. Preheat broiler.

2. Combine turkey, green onions, parsley, wine, Italian seasoning, salt and black pepper in large bowl; mix well. Shape turkey mixture into 4 (¾-inch-thick) burgers.

3. Spray rack of broiler pan with nonstick cooking spray; place burgers on rack. Broil burgers 4 inches from heat 5 to 6 minutes per side or until no longer pink in center. Serve on whole wheat buns with lettuce, grilled pineapple slices and bell pepper strips, if desired.   *Makes 4 servings*

black and white chili

   Nonstick cooking spray
   1 pound chicken tenders, cut into ¾-inch pieces
   1 cup coarsely chopped onion
   1 can (15½ ounces) Great Northern beans, rinsed and drained
   1 can (15 ounces) black beans, rinsed and drained
   1 can (14½ ounces) Mexican-style stewed tomatoes, undrained
   2 tablespoons Texas-style chili powder seasoning mix

1. Spray large saucepan with cooking spray; heat over medium heat until hot. Add chicken and onion; cook and stir over medium to medium-high heat 5 to 8 minutes or until chicken is browned.

2. Stir beans, tomatoes with juice and seasoning mix into saucepan; bring to a boil. Reduce heat to low; simmer, uncovered, 10 minutes.   *Makes 6 servings*

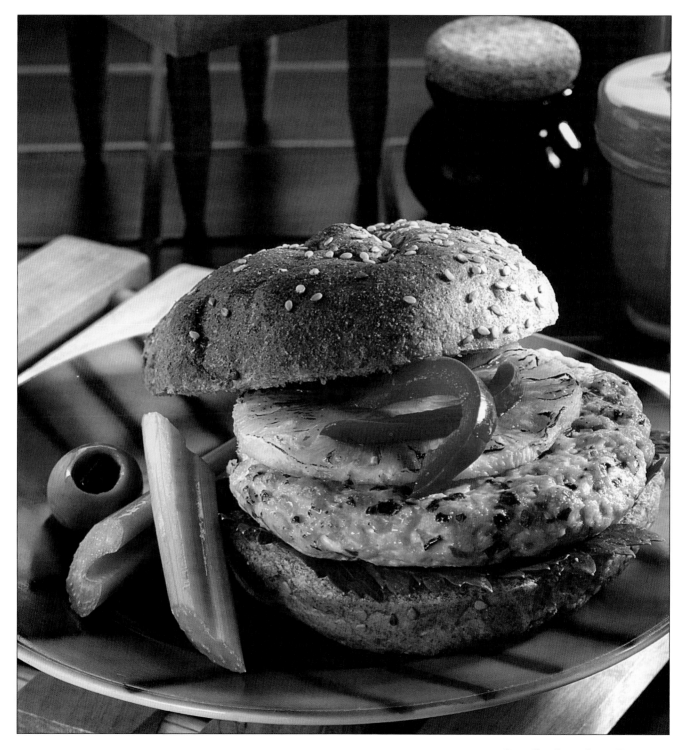

broiled turkey burger

main dishes

browned pork chops with gravy

nutrients per serving:

1 pork chop with ½ cup noodles and ¼ of gravy

Calories: 315

Carbohydrate: 30 g

Dietary Fiber: 2 g

Total Fat: 10 g

Calories From Fat: 29%

Saturated Fat: 3 g

Cholesterol: 67 mg

Sodium: 296 mg

Protein: 25 g

Exchanges: 1½ Starch, 1 Vegetable, 3 Lean Meat

4 boneless pork loin chops (about ¾ pound)
½ teaspoon dried sage leaves
½ teaspoon dried marjoram leaves
¼ teaspoon black pepper
⅛ teaspoon salt
Nonstick olive oil cooking spray
¼ cup coarsely chopped onion
1 clove garlic, minced
1 cup sliced mushrooms
¾ cup beef broth
⅓ cup fat-free sour cream
1 tablespoon all-purpose flour
1 teaspoon Dijon mustard
2 cups hot cooked noodles
Snipped parsley (optional)

1. Trim fat from chops. Combine sage, marjoram, pepper and salt in small bowl. Rub on both sides of chops. Spray large nonstick skillet with cooking spray; heat over medium heat. Place chops in skillet. Cook 5 minutes, turning once, or until chops are just barely pink. Remove chops from skillet; keep warm.

2. Add onion and garlic to skillet; cook and stir 2 minutes. Add mushrooms and broth. Bring to a boil. Reduce heat; simmer, covered, 3 to 4 minutes or until mushrooms are tender.

3. Whisk together sour cream, flour and mustard in medium bowl. Whisk in about 3 tablespoons broth mixture from skillet. Stir sour cream mixture into skillet. Cook, stirring constantly, until mixture comes to a boil. Serve over pork chops and noodles. Sprinkle with parsley, if desired. *Makes 4 servings*

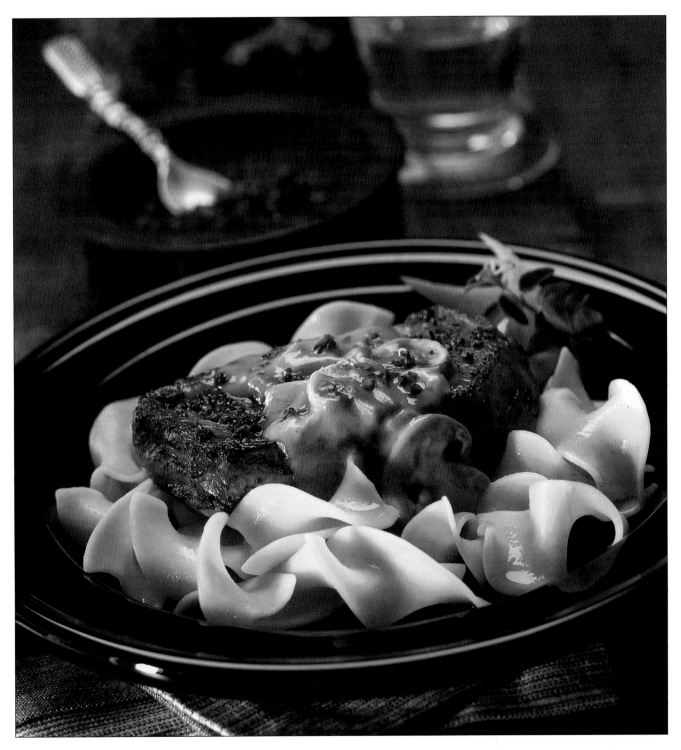

browned pork chop with gravy

lemon-dijon chicken with potatoes

nutrients per serving:

⅙ of total recipe

Calories: 294

Carbohydrate: 26 g

Dietary Fiber: 3 g

Total Fat: 9 g

Calories From Fat: 27%

Saturated Fat: 2 g

Cholesterol: 84 mg

Sodium: 348 mg

Protein: 30 g

Exchanges: 2 Starch, 3 Lean Meat

2 medium lemons
½ cup chopped fresh parsley
2 tablespoons Dijon mustard
4 cloves garlic, minced
2 teaspoons extra-virgin olive oil
1 teaspoon dried rosemary leaves, crushed
¾ teaspoon black pepper
½ teaspoon salt
1 whole chicken (about 3½ pounds)
1½ pounds small red potatoes, cut into halves

1. Preheat oven to 350°F.

2. Squeeze 3 tablespoons juice from lemons; reserve squeezed lemon halves. Combine parsley, lemon juice, mustard, garlic, oil, rosemary, pepper and salt in small bowl; blend well. Reserve 2 tablespoons mixture.

3. Place chicken on rack in baking pan. Gently slide fingers between skin and meat of chicken breasts and drumsticks to separate skin from meat, being careful not to tear skin. Spoon parsley mixture between skin and meat. (Secure breast skin with toothpicks, if necessary.) Discard any remaining parsley mixture (not reserved 2 tablespoons). Place lemon halves in cavity of chicken. Bake 30 minutes.

4. Meanwhile, toss potatoes with reserved parsley mixture until coated. Arrange potatoes around chicken; bake 1 hour or until juices in chicken run clear and thermometer inserted into thickest part of thigh registers 180°F. Remove chicken from oven; let stand 10 minutes. Remove skin; discard. Slice chicken. Sprinkle any accumulated parsley mixture from pan over chicken and potatoes.
Makes 6 servings

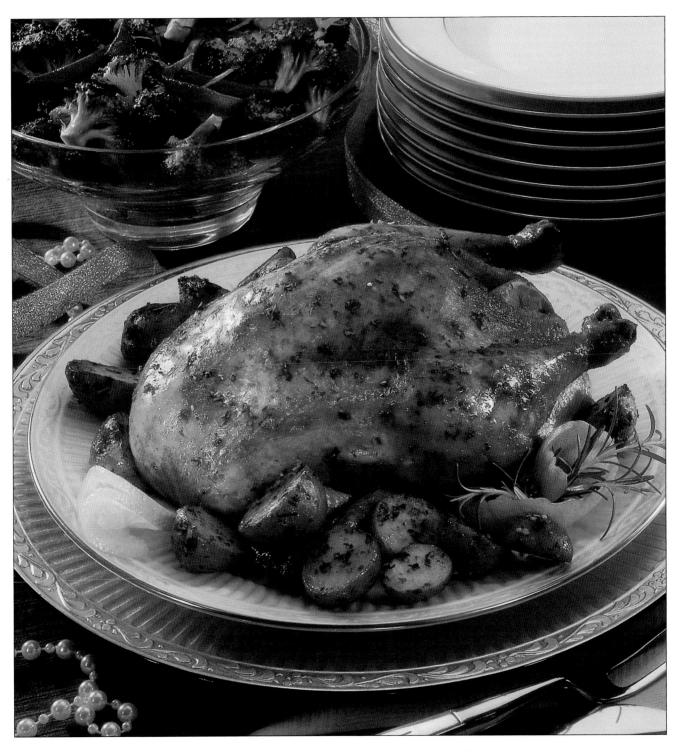

lemon-dijon chicken with potatoes

teriyaki salmon with asian slaw

nutrients per serving:

1 salmon fillet with about 2 cups slaw
Calories: 354
Carbohydrate: 32 g
Dietary Fiber: 5 g
Total Fat: 11 g
Calories From Fat: 28%
Saturated Fat: 2 g
Cholesterol: 75 mg
Sodium: 730 mg
Protein: 32 g

Exchanges: 1 Starch, 4 Vegetable, 3½ Lean Meat

4 tablespoons light teriyaki sauce, divided
2 (5- to 6-ounce) boneless salmon fillets with skin (1 inch thick)
2½ cups packaged coleslaw mix
1 cup fresh or frozen snow peas, cut lengthwise into thin strips
½ cup thinly sliced radishes
2 tablespoons orange marmalade
1 teaspoon dark sesame oil

1. Preheat broiler or prepare grill for direct cooking. Spoon 2 tablespoons teriyaki sauce over fleshy sides of salmon. Let stand while preparing vegetable mixture.

2. Combine coleslaw mix, snow peas and radishes in large bowl. Combine remaining 2 tablespoons teriyaki sauce, marmalade and sesame oil in small bowl. Add to coleslaw mixture; toss well.

3. Broil salmon 4 to 5 inches from heat source or grill, flesh side down, over medium coals, without turning, 6 to 10 minutes or until center is opaque.

4. Transfer coleslaw mixture to serving plates; top with salmon.

Makes 2 servings

cajun grilled chicken

nutrients per serving:

1 (4-ounce) grilled chicken breast
Calories: 148
Carbohydrate: 6 g
Dietary Fiber: 1 g
Total Fat: 2 g
Calories From Fat: 11%
Saturated Fat: <1 g
Cholesterol: 66 mg
Sodium: 61 mg
Protein: 27 g

Exchanges: ½ Starch, 2½ Lean Meat

4 boneless skinless chicken breast halves
2 tablespoons lemon juice
3 tablespoons MRS. DASH® Extra Spicy Seasoning
2 tablespoons paprika
1 tablespoon brown sugar
Cooking spray

Preheat grill to medium-high. With a sharp knife, slash each piece of chicken in 2 or 3 places with ¼-inch-deep cuts. In a bowl, combine chicken and lemon juice, turning the chicken until it is thoroughly coated. Set aside. In separate bowl, mix Mrs. Dash Extra Spicy Seasoning, paprika and brown sugar. Take each piece of chicken and roll in the spice mixture until well coated. Spray grill with cooking spray and place seasoned chicken breasts on the grill. Cook 5 minutes and turn. Cook 5 minutes more or until juices run clear when a skewer is inserted. Serve immediately.

Makes 4 servings

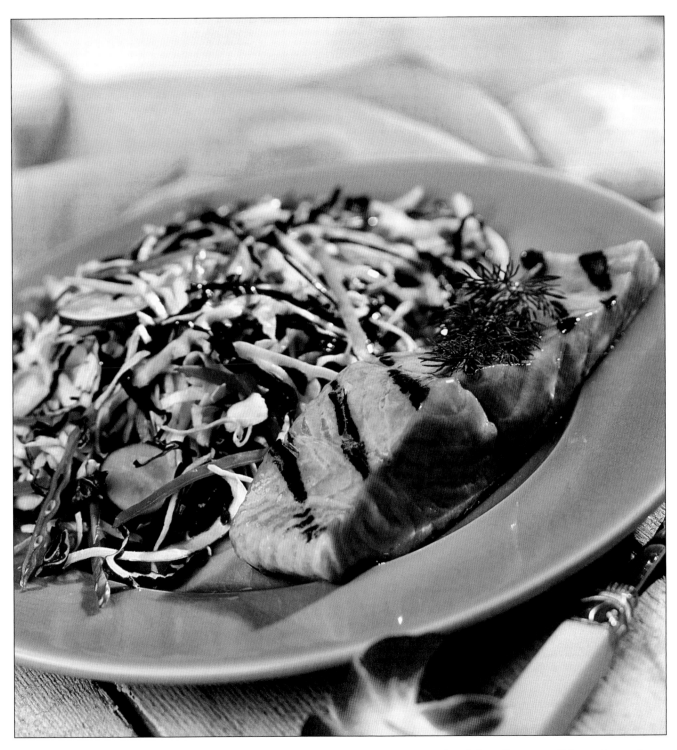

teriyaki salmon with asian slaw

lamb chops with cranberry-pear chutney

nutrients per
serving:
1 lamb chop with
¼ cup chutney
Calories: 260
Carbohydrate: 24 g
Dietary Fiber: 2 g
Total Fat: 8 g
Calories From Fat: 28%
Saturated Fat: 3 g
Cholesterol: 71 mg
Sodium: 293 mg
Protein: 22 g
Exchanges: 1½ Fruit,
3 Lean Meat

Chutney
  ½ **cup water**
  ¼ **cup dried cranberries**
  ¼ **cup dried apricots, cut into quarters**
  ¼ **cup no-sugar-added raspberry spread**
  1 **tablespoon red wine vinegar**
  ¼ **teaspoon ground cinnamon**
  ⅛ **teaspoon salt**
  1 **medium pear, peeled and cut into ½-inch pieces**
  ½ **teaspoon vanilla**

Lamb
  4 **bone-in lamb loin chops (about 5 ounces each)**
  2 **cloves garlic, minced**
  ¼ **teaspoon dried rosemary leaves, crushed**
  ¼ **teaspoon salt**
    Black pepper

1. Preheat broiler. For chutney, combine water, cranberries, apricots, raspberry spread, vinegar, cinnamon and ⅛ teaspoon salt in medium saucepan; bring to a boil over high heat. Reduce heat to medium-low; simmer, uncovered, 12 minutes or until mixture is thickened. Remove from heat; stir in pear and vanilla.

2. For lamb, rub both sides of chops with garlic. Sprinkle with rosemary, ¼ teaspoon salt and pepper. Coat broiler pan and rack with nonstick cooking spray. Place lamb on rack; broil at least 5 inches from heat source 7 minutes; turn and broil 7 minutes more or until of desired doneness. Serve lamb chops with chutney. *Makes 4 servings*

lamb chop with cranberry-pear chutney

nutrients per serving:

1 lasagna piece

Calories: 287
Carbohydrate: 33 g
Dietary Fiber: 3 g
Total Fat: 7 g
Calories From Fat: 22%
Saturated Fat: 4 g
Cholesterol: 22 mg
Sodium: 568 mg
Protein: 23 g

Exchanges: 1 Starch, 3 Vegetable, 2 Lean Meat, ½ Fat

fresh vegetable lasagna

8 ounces uncooked lasagna noodles
1 package (10 ounces) frozen chopped spinach, thawed and well drained
1 cup shredded carrots
½ cup sliced green onions
½ cup sliced red bell pepper
¼ cup chopped fresh parsley
½ teaspoon black pepper
1½ cups low-fat (1%) cottage cheese
1 cup buttermilk
½ cup plain nonfat yogurt
2 egg whites
1 cup sliced mushrooms
1 can (14 ounces) artichoke hearts, drained and chopped
2 cups (8 ounces) shredded part-skim mozzarella cheese, divided
¼ cup freshly grated Parmesan cheese

1. Cook pasta according to package directions, omitting salt; drain. Rinse under cold water; drain well. Set aside.

2. Preheat oven to 375°F. Pat spinach with paper towels to remove excess moisture. Combine spinach, carrots, green onions, bell pepper, parsley and black pepper in large bowl; set aside.

3. Combine cottage cheese, buttermilk, yogurt and egg whites in food processor or blender. Cover; process until smooth.

4. Spray 13×9-inch baking pan with nonstick cooking spray. Arrange third of lasagna noodles in bottom of pan. Spread with half of cottage cheese mixture, half of vegetable mixture, half of mushrooms, half of artichokes and ¾ cup mozzarella. Repeat layers, ending with noodles. Sprinkle with remaining ½ cup mozzarella and Parmesan.

5. Cover; bake 30 minutes. Remove cover; continue baking 20 minutes or until bubbly and heated through. Remove from oven; let stand 10 minutes. Cut into 8 pieces to serve.

Makes 8 servings

fresh vegetable lasagna

broccoli-fish roll-ups

1 can (10¾ ounces) cream of broccoli soup, undiluted
½ cup fat-free (skim) milk
2 cups uncooked seasoned stuffing crumbs
4 flounder fillets (about 3 ounces each)
1 box (10 ounces) frozen broccoli spears, thawed
Paprika

1. Preheat oven to 375°F. Spray 9×9-inch baking pan with nonstick cooking spray. Combine soup and milk in medium bowl. Reserve ½ cup soup mixture.

2. Combine stuffing crumbs and remaining soup mixture in medium bowl; pat into prepared pan.

3. Place fish on clean work surface. Arrange 1 broccoli spear crosswise across narrow end of 1 fillet. Starting at narrow end, gently roll up fish. Place over stuffing mixture, seam side down. Repeat with remaining fish and broccoli.

4. Arrange any remaining broccoli spears over stuffing mixture. Spoon reserved ½ cup soup mixture over broccoli-fish roll-ups. Sprinkle with paprika. Bake 20 minutes or until fish flakes easily when tested with fork. *Makes 4 servings*

fajita-seasoned grilled chicken

2 boneless skinless chicken breasts (about 4 ounces each)
1 bunch green onions, ends trimmed
1 tablespoon olive oil
2 teaspoons fajita seasoning mix

1. Preheat grill for direct cooking.

2. Brush chicken and green onions with oil. Sprinkle both sides of chicken breasts with seasoning mix. Grill chicken and onions 6 to 8 minutes or until chicken is no longer pink in center. Serve chicken with onions. *Makes 2 servings*

broccoli-fish roll-ups

oven-fried chicken

2 boneless skinless chicken breasts (about 4 ounces each)
4 small skinless chicken drumsticks (about 2½ ounces each)
3 tablespoons all-purpose flour
½ teaspoon poultry seasoning
¼ teaspoon garlic salt
¼ teaspoon black pepper
1½ cups cornflakes, crushed
1 tablespoon dried parsley flakes
1 egg white
1 tablespoon water
Nonstick cooking spray

1. Preheat oven to 375°F. Rinse chicken; pat dry with paper towels. Trim fat from chicken; discard.

2. Combine flour, poultry seasoning, garlic salt and pepper in large resealable plastic food storage bag. Combine cornflake crumbs and parsley in small shallow bowl. Whisk together egg white and water in small bowl.

3. Add chicken to flour mixture, one or two pieces at a time. Seal bag; shake until chicken is well coated. Remove chicken from bag, shaking off excess flour. Dip into egg white mixture, coating all sides. Roll in crumb mixture. Place in shallow baking pan. Repeat with remaining chicken, flour mixture, egg white and crumb mixture.

4. Lightly spray chicken pieces with cooking spray. Bake breasts 18 to 20 minutes or until no longer pink in center. Bake drumsticks about 25 minutes or until juices run clear.

Makes 4 servings

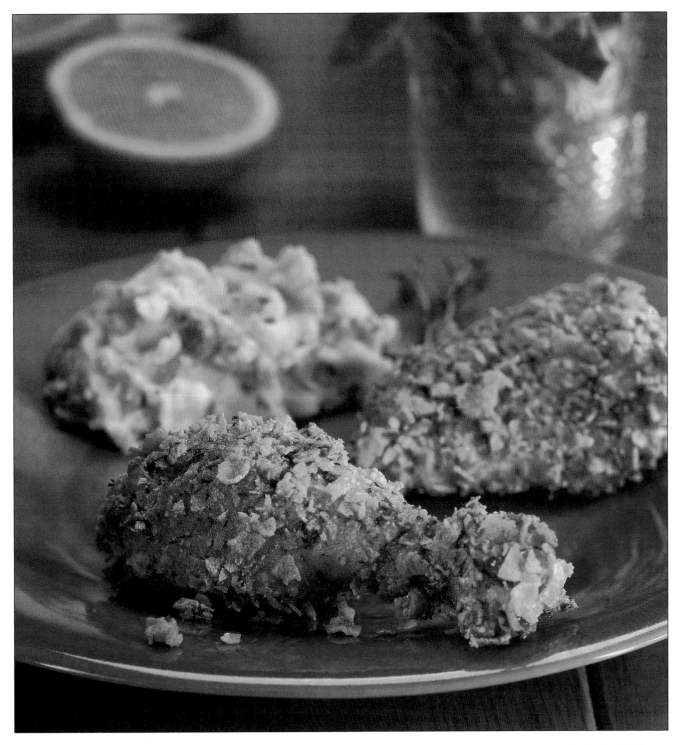

oven-fried chicken

nutrients per serving:

¹⁄₁₀ of total recipe

Calories: 284

Carbohydrate: 18 g

Dietary Fiber: 1 g

Total Fat: 8 g

Calories From Fat: 26%

Saturated Fat: 3 g

Cholesterol: 70 mg

Sodium: 82 mg

Protein: 31 g

Exchanges: 1 Fruit, 4 Lean Meat

pork roast with dried cranberries and apricots

      1 center-cut pork loin roast (about 3½ pounds)
  1½ cups cranberry-apple juice, divided
      1 cup chardonnay or other dry white wine
  1½ teaspoons ground ginger
      1 teaspoon ground cardamom
      2 tablespoons apricot preserves
   ¼ cup water
      1 tablespoon plus 1 teaspoon cornstarch
   ½ cup dried cranberries
   ½ cup chopped dried apricots
      2 tablespoons golden raisins

1. Place pork roast in large resealable plastic food storage bag. Combine 1 cup cranberry-apple juice, chardonnay, ginger and cardamom in medium bowl. Pour over roast, turning to coat. Seal bag. Marinate in refrigerator 4 hours or overnight, turning several times.

2. Preheat oven to 350°F. Remove roast from marinade; reserve marinade. Place roast in roasting pan. Pour marinade over roast. Bake, loosely covered with foil, 1 hour. Remove foil; continue baking 30 minutes or until internal temperature of roast reaches 165°F when tested with meat thermometer inserted into thickest part of roast. Transfer roast to cutting board; cover with foil. Internal temperature will continue to rise 5°F to 10°F during stand time.

3. Measure juices from pan. Add enough remaining cranberry-apple juice to equal 1½ cups. Combine juices and apricot preserves in small saucepan. Stir water into cornstarch in small bowl until smooth; stir into juice mixture. Bring to a boil over medium heat. Cook until thickened, stirring frequently. Add dried cranberries, apricots and raisins; cook 2 minutes. Remove from heat. Cut roast into thin slices. Drizzle some sauce over roast; serve with remaining sauce. Garnish, if desired.

Makes 10 servings

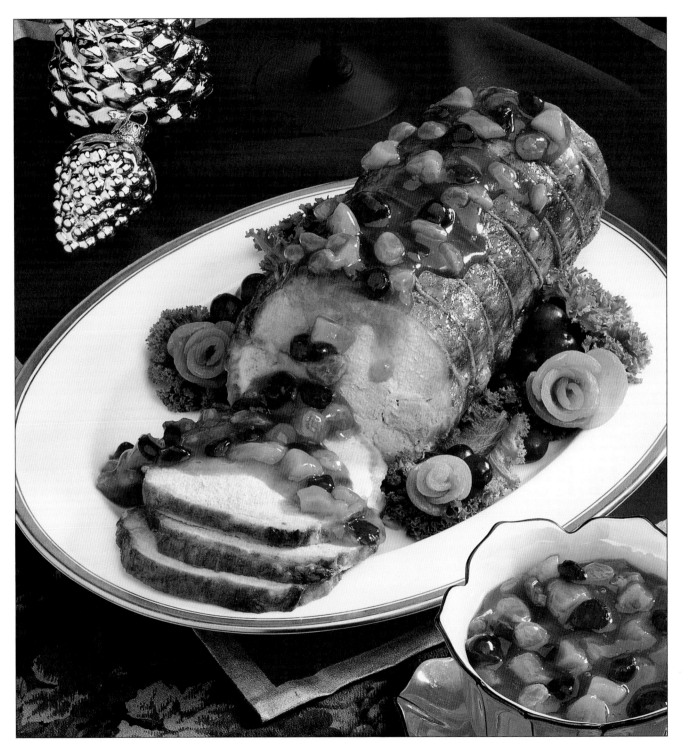

pork roast with dried cranberries and apricots

broccoli, scallop and linguine toss

nutrients per serving:
¼ of total recipe (with 1 cup linguine)
Calories: 248
Carbohydrate: 33 g
Dietary Fiber: 4 g
Total Fat: 4 g
Calories From Fat: 13%
Saturated Fat: 1 g
Cholesterol: 33 mg
Sodium: 309 mg
Protein: 22 g

Exchanges: 1 Starch, ½ Fruit, 1½ Vegetable, 2 Lean Meat

¾ pound uncooked fresh or frozen scallops
2 medium onions, cut in half lengthwise and sliced
1 cup apple juice
2 tablespoons dry white wine
2 cloves garlic, minced
2 teaspoons dried marjoram leaves
1 teaspoon dried basil leaves
¼ teaspoon black pepper
3 cups broccoli florets
¼ cup water
1 tablespoon plus 1 teaspoon cornstarch
1½ cups chopped seeded fresh tomatoes
¼ cup grated Parmesan cheese
4 cups hot cooked linguine

1. Cut large scallops into 1-inch pieces; set aside.

2. Combine onions, apple juice, wine, garlic, marjoram, basil and pepper in large skillet; bring to a boil over high heat. Add broccoli; return to a boil. Reduce heat to medium-low. Cover; simmer 7 minutes. Add scallops; return to a boil. Reduce heat. Cover; simmer 1 to 2 minutes or until scallops are opaque. Remove scallops and vegetables; set aside.

3. Combine water and cornstarch in small bowl; stir into mixture in skillet. Cook and stir over medium heat until mixture boils and thickens. Cook and stir 2 minutes more. Stir in tomatoes and cheese; heat through. Return scallops and vegetables to skillet; heat through. Toss mixture with linguine.

Makes 4 servings

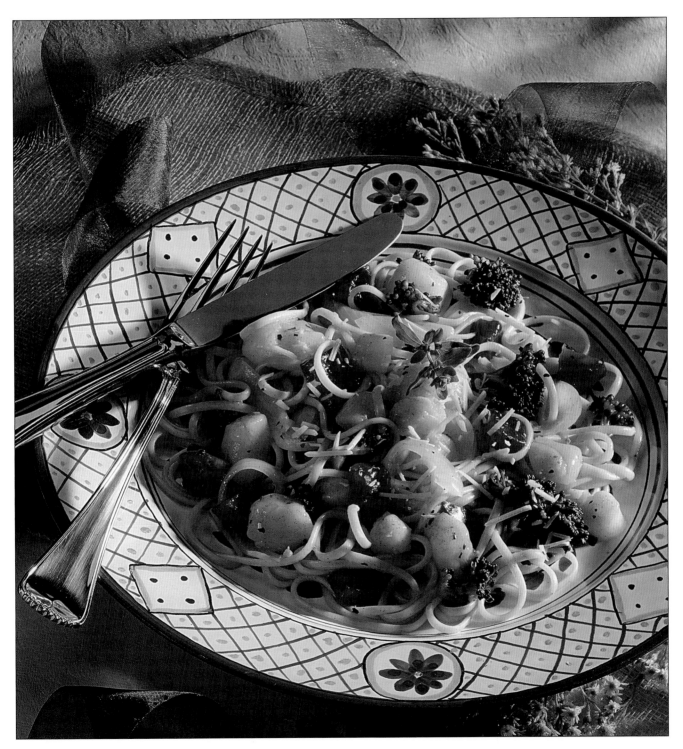

broccoli, scallop and linguine toss

sassy chicken & peppers

2 teaspoons Mexican seasoning*
2 boneless skinless chicken breasts (about 4 ounces each)
2 teaspoons vegetable oil
1 small red onion, sliced
½ medium red bell pepper, cut into thin strips
½ medium yellow or green bell pepper, cut into long, thin strips
¼ cup chunky salsa or chipotle salsa
1 tablespoon lime juice
Lime wedges, for garnish (optional)

If Mexican seasoning is not available, substitute 1 teaspoon chili powder, ½ teaspoon ground cumin, ½ teaspoon salt and ⅛ teaspoon ground red pepper.

1. Sprinkle seasoning over both sides of chicken.

2. Heat oil in large nonstick skillet over medium heat. Add onion; cook 3 minutes, stirring occasionally.

3. Add bell pepper strips; cook 3 minutes, stirring occasionally.

4. Push vegetables to edge of skillet. Add chicken to skillet. Cook 5 minutes; turn. Stir salsa and lime juice into vegetables. Continue to cook 4 minutes or until chicken is no longer pink in center and vegetables are tender.

5. Transfer chicken to serving plates; top with vegetable mixture. Garnish with lime wedges, if desired.

Makes 2 servings

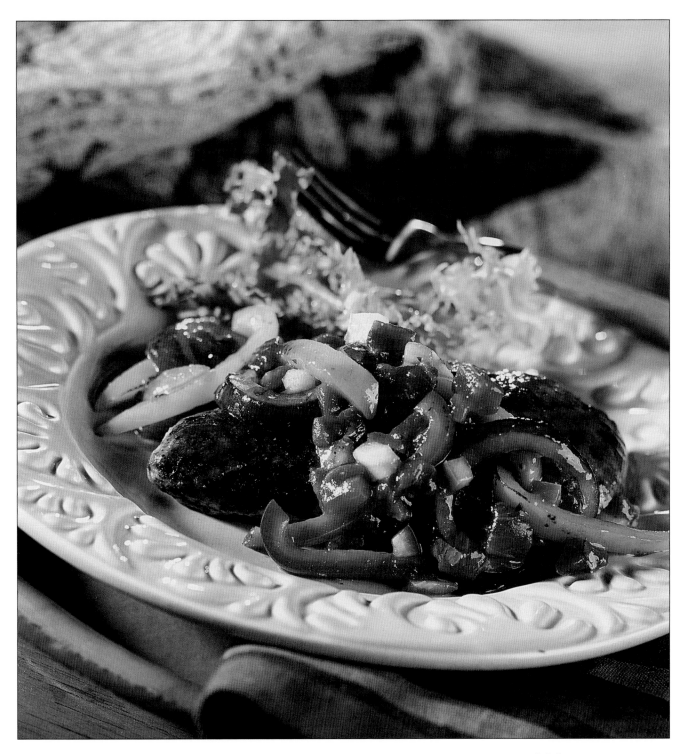

sassy chicken & peppers

cannelloni with tomato-eggplant sauce

1 package (10 ounces) fresh spinach, stemmed
1 cup fat-free ricotta cheese
4 egg whites, beaten
¼ cup grated Parmesan cheese
2 tablespoons finely chopped fresh parsley
½ teaspoon salt (optional)
8 manicotti shells (about 4 ounces uncooked),
**   cooked (without added salt) and cooled**
Tomato-Eggplant Sauce (recipe follows)
1 cup (4 ounces) shredded reduced-fat mozzarella cheese

1. Preheat oven to 350°F. Wash spinach; do not pat dry. Place spinach in large saucepan; cook, covered, over medium-high heat 3 to 5 minutes or until spinach is wilted. Cool slightly; drain. Chop finely.

2. Combine ricotta cheese, spinach, egg whites, Parmesan cheese, parsley and salt, if desired, in large bowl; mix well. Spoon mixture into cooked manicotti shells; arrange in 13×9-inch baking pan. Spoon Tomato-Eggplant Sauce over manicotti; sprinkle with mozzarella cheese. Bake, uncovered, 25 to 30 minutes or until hot and bubbly.

Makes 4 servings

tomato-eggplant sauce

Nonstick olive oil cooking spray
1 small eggplant, coarsely chopped
½ cup chopped onion
2 cloves garlic, minced
½ teaspoon dried tarragon leaves
¼ teaspoon dried thyme leaves
1 can (16 ounces) no-salt-added whole tomatoes, undrained,
**   coarsely chopped**

1. Spray large skillet with cooking spray; heat over medium heat until hot. Add eggplant, onion, garlic, tarragon and thyme; cook and stir about 5 minutes or until vegetables are tender.

2. Stir in tomatoes with juice; bring to a boil. Reduce heat; simmer, uncovered, 3 to 4 minutes.

Makes about 2½ cups

cannelloni with tomato-eggplant sauce

beef tenderloin with roasted vegetables

nutrients per serving:

¹/₁₀ of total recipe

Calories: 326
Carbohydrate: 24 g
Dietary Fiber: 1 g
Total Fat: 10 g
Calories From Fat: 26%
Saturated Fat: 3 g
Cholesterol: 71 mg
Sodium: 546 mg
Protein: 34 g

Exchanges: 1 Starch,
1½ Vegetable,
4 Lean Meat

1 beef tenderloin roast (about 3 pounds), trimmed of fat
½ cup chardonnay or other dry white wine
½ cup reduced-sodium soy sauce
2 cloves garlic, sliced
1 tablespoon fresh rosemary
1 tablespoon Dijon mustard
1 teaspoon dry mustard
1 pound small red or white potatoes, cut into 1-inch pieces
1 pound brussels sprouts
1 package (12 ounces) baby carrots
Fresh rosemary, for garnish (optional)

1. Place roast in large resealable plastic food storage bag. Combine wine, soy sauce, garlic, rosemary, Dijon mustard and dry mustard in small bowl. Pour over roast. Seal bag; turn to coat. Marinate in refrigerator 4 to 12 hours, turning several times.

2. Preheat oven to 425°F. Spray 13×9-inch baking pan with nonstick cooking spray. Place potatoes, brussels sprouts and carrots in pan. Remove roast from marinade. Pour marinade over vegetables; toss to coat well. Cover vegetables with foil; bake 30 minutes. Stir.

3. Place tenderloin on vegetables. Roast, uncovered, 35 to 45 minutes or until internal temperature of roast reaches 135°F for medium-rare to 150°F for medium when tested with meat thermometer inserted into thickest part of roast.

4. Transfer roast to cutting board; cover with foil. Let stand 10 to 15 minutes before carving. (Internal temperature will continue to rise 5°F to 10°F during stand time.)

5. Stir vegetables; test for doneness. Continue to bake if not tender. Slice tenderloin; arrange on serving platter with roasted vegetables. Garnish with fresh rosemary, if desired.   *Makes 10 servings*

beef tenderloin with roasted vegetables

chicken with spinach and celery hash

1 package (16 ounces) refrigerated pre-cooked fat-free hash browns
1 package (8 ounces) ready-to-use celery sticks, thinly sliced
3 teaspoons olive oil, divided
12 chicken tenders (about 1 pound)
½ teaspoon dried thyme leaves
¼ teaspoon ground white pepper
2 packages (5 ounces each) ready-to-use baby spinach
¼ cup water

1. Combine hash browns and celery in medium bowl.

2. Heat 1½ teaspoons oil in large nonstick skillet over medium-high heat. Add hash brown mixture; cook about 10 minutes, stirring and turning occasionally, or until mixture begins to brown. Reduce heat; cook 10 minutes or until browned.

3. Heat remaining 1½ teaspoons oil in 12-inch nonstick skillet over medium-high heat until hot. Add chicken tenders. Sprinkle with thyme and pepper. Cook about 5 minutes, turning once, or until no longer pink in center. Remove from skillet; keep warm.

4. Add spinach and water to same skillet. Cover; cook about 3 minutes, stirring once.

5. To serve, divide spinach and hash brown mixture evenly among 4 plates. Top each with 3 chicken tenders. *Makes 4 servings*

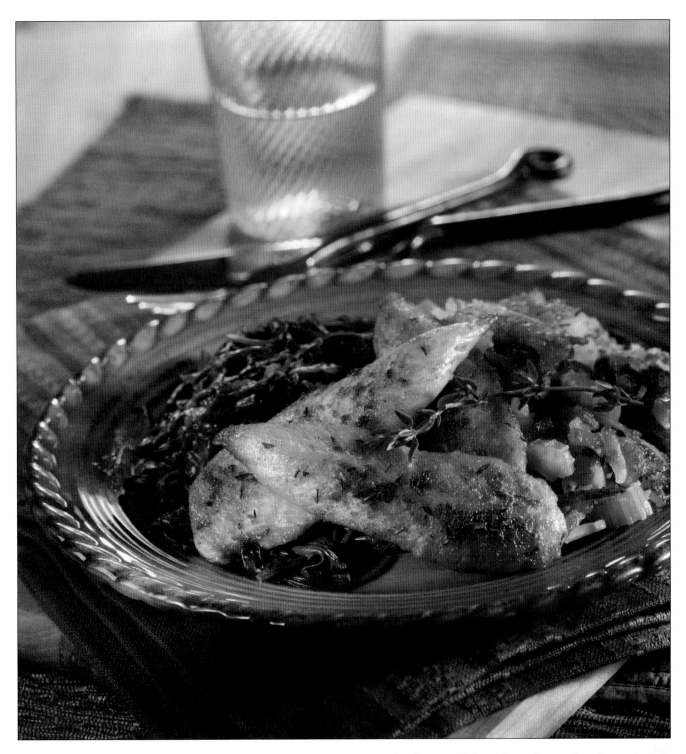

chicken with spinach and celery hash

sweet and sour stir-fry

1 tablespoon vegetable oil
1 pound boneless skinless chicken breasts, cut into 3-inch strips
1 can (8 ounces) sliced water chestnuts, drained
1 cup red bell pepper strips
¼ cup chopped onion
2 tablespoons cornstarch
2 tablespoons soy sauce
1 tablespoon white vinegar
1 can (8 ounces) pineapple chunks, packed in juice, undrained
¼ teaspoon ground ginger
¼ teaspoon salt
¼ cup EQUAL® SPOONFUL*
1 package (6 ounces) frozen pea pods

*May substitute 6 packets Equal® sweetener.

● Heat oil in wok or skillet. Add chicken; cook and stir 5 to 6 minutes or until chicken is no longer pink. Remove and set aside. Add water chestnuts, pepper and onion to wok; cook 3 to 4 minutes or until vegetables are tender, stirring constantly.

● Combine cornstarch, soy sauce and vinegar in small bowl; stir to dissolve cornstarch. Add pineapple with juice, ginger and salt. Add to vegetable mixture; cook 2 to 3 minutes or until sauce thickens, stirring constantly.

● Stir in Equal® Spoonful. Add pea pods and chicken; cook until pea pods and chicken are heated through, 2 to 3 minutes.   *Makes 4 servings*

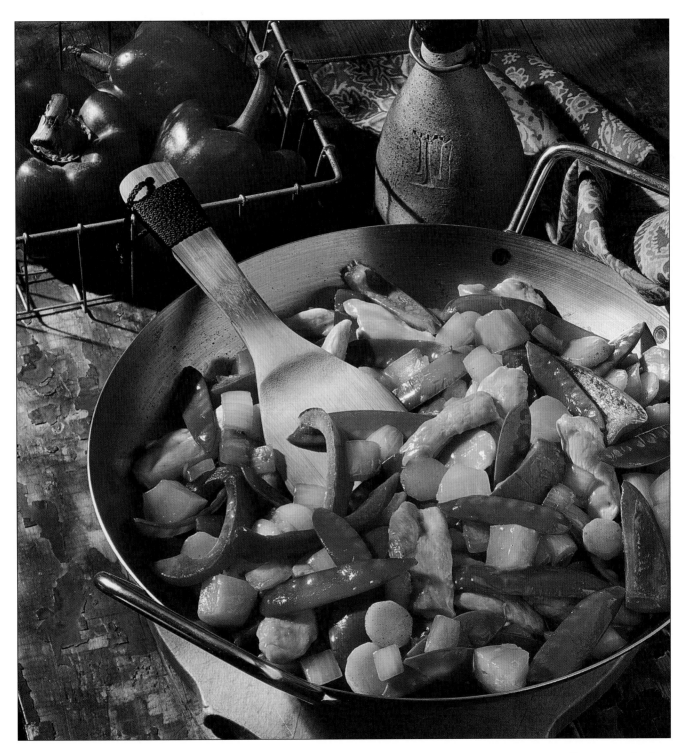

sweet and sour stir-fry

side dishes

roasted red pepper & tomato casserole

    1 jar (12 ounces) roasted red peppers, drained
1½ teaspoons red wine vinegar
    1 teaspoon olive oil
    1 clove garlic, minced
    ¼ teaspoon salt
    ¼ teaspoon black pepper
    ⅓ cup grated Parmesan cheese, divided
    3 medium fresh tomatoes (about 1½ pounds), sliced
    ½ cup (about 1 ounce) herb-flavored croutons, crushed

Microwave Directions

1. Combine red peppers, vinegar, oil, garlic, salt and black pepper in food processor. Cover; process, using on/off pulsing action, 1 minute or until slightly chunky. Reserve 2 tablespoons cheese for garnish. Stir remaining cheese into red pepper mixture.

2. Arrange tomato slices in 8-inch round microwavable baking dish; microwave at HIGH 1 minute. Spoon red pepper mixture on top; microwave at HIGH 2 to 3 minutes or until tomatoes are slightly softened.

3. Sprinkle with reserved 2 tablespoons cheese and croutons. Garnish, if desired.

Makes 6 servings

cool and creamy pea salad with cucumbers and red onion

    2 tablespoons finely chopped red onion
    1 tablespoon reduced-fat mayonnaise
    ⅛ teaspoon salt
    ⅛ teaspoon black pepper
    ½ cup frozen green peas, thawed
    ¼ cup diced red bell pepper
    ¼ cup diced cucumber

1. Combine onion, mayonnaise, salt and black pepper in medium bowl; stir until well blended.

2. Add remaining ingredients; toss gently to coat.

Makes 2 servings

roasted red pepper & tomato casserole

zucchini delight

nutrients per serving:

⅙ of total recipe

Calories: 92
Carbohydrate: 18 g
Dietary Fiber: 3 g
Total Fat: 2 g
Calories From Fat: 14%
Saturated Fat: <1 g
Cholesterol: 1 mg
Sodium: 426 mg
Protein: 4 g

Exchanges: 3½ Vegetable

1 can (10¾ ounces) reduced-fat condensed tomato soup, undiluted
1 tablespoon lemon juice
1 teaspoon sugar
2 cloves garlic, minced
½ teaspoon salt
6 cups ½-inch zucchini slices
1 cup thinly sliced onion
1 cup coarsely chopped green bell pepper
1 cup sliced mushrooms
2 tablespoons grated Parmesan cheese

Combine soup, lemon juice, sugar, garlic and salt in large saucepan; mix well. Add zucchini, onion, bell pepper and mushrooms; mix well. Bring to a boil; reduce heat. Cover; cook 20 to 25 minutes or until vegetables are crisp-tender, stirring occasionally. Sprinkle with cheese before serving.   *Makes 6 servings*

jalapeño coleslaw

nutrients per serving:

about 1 cup coleslaw

Calories: 47
Carbohydrate: 12 g
Dietary Fiber: 2 g
Total Fat: <1 g
Calories From Fat: 4%
Saturated Fat: <1 g
Cholesterol: 0 mg
Sodium: 304 mg
Protein: 1 g

Exchanges: ½ Starch,
1 Vegetable

6 cups shredded cabbage or coleslaw mix
2 medium fresh tomatoes, seeded and chopped
6 green onions, coarsely chopped
2 jalapeño peppers,* finely chopped
¼ cup cider vinegar
3 tablespoons honey
1 teaspoon salt

*Jalapeño peppers can sting and irritate the skin. Wear rubber gloves when handling peppers and do not touch eyes. Wash hands after handling peppers.

1. Combine cabbage, tomatoes, green onions, jalapeño peppers, vinegar, honey and salt in serving bowl; mix well. Cover; chill at least 2 hours before serving.

2. Stir well immediately before serving.   *Makes 8 servings*

Tip: For a milder coleslaw, discard the seeds and veins when chopping the jalapeños, since this is where much of the heat of the peppers is stored.

zucchini delight

nutrients per serving:

1 triangle

Calories: 62
Carbohydrate: 9 g
Dietary Fiber: <1 g
Total Fat: 2 g
Calories From Fat: 26%
Saturated Fat: 1 g
Cholesterol: 6 mg
Sodium: 142 mg
Protein: 3 g

Exchanges: 1 Starch

polenta triangles

½ cup uncooked yellow corn grits
1 ½ cups fat-free reduced-sodium chicken broth, divided
 2 cloves garlic, minced
½ cup (2 ounces) crumbled feta cheese
 1 red bell pepper, roasted,* peeled and finely chopped

*Place pepper on foil-lined broiler pan; broil 15 minutes or until blackened on all sides, turning every 5 minutes. Place pepper in paper bag. Cose bag; let stand 15 minutes before peeling.

1. Combine grits and ½ cup chicken broth in small bowl; mix well. Set aside. Pour remaining 1 cup broth into large heavy saucepan; bring to a boil. Add garlic and moistened grits; mix well. Return to a boil. Reduce heat to low. Cover; cook 20 minutes. Remove from heat; add feta cheese. Stir until cheese is completely melted. Add roasted bell pepper; mix well.

2. Spray 8-inch square pan with nonstick cooking spray. Spoon grits mixture into prepared pan. With wet fingertips, press grits evenly into pan. Refrigerate until cold.

3. Spray grid with nonstick cooking spray. Prepare grill for direct cooking. Turn polenta out onto cutting board; cut into 4 (2-inch) squares. Cut each square diagonally into 2 triangles.

4. Place polenta triangles on grid. Grill over medium-high heat 1 minute or until bottoms are lightly browned. Turn triangles over; grill until browned and crisp. Serve warm or at room temperature. *Makes 8 servings*

nutrients per serving:

⅒ of total recipe

Calories: 64
Carbohydrate: 6 g
Dietary Fiber: 2 g
Total Fat: 5 g
Calories From Fat: 61%
Saturated Fat: <1 g
Cholesterol: 0 mg
Sodium: 14 mg
Protein: 7 g

Exchanges: 1 Vegetable, 1 Fat

collard greens

4 bunches collard greens, stemmed, washed and torn into bite-size pieces
2 cups water
½ medium red bell pepper, cored, seeded and cut into strips
⅓ medium green bell pepper, cored, seeded and cut into strips
¼ cup olive oil
¼ teaspoon salt
¼ teaspoon black pepper

Place all ingredients in large saucepan; bring to a boil. Reduce heat; simmer 1 to 1 ½ hours or until tender. *Makes 10 servings*

polenta triangles

roasted butternut squash

Nonstick cooking spray
1 pound butternut squash, peeled and cut into 1-inch cubes (about 4 cups)
2 medium onions, coarsely chopped
8 ounces carrots, peeled and cut into ½-inch diagonal slices (about 2 cups)
1 tablespoon dark brown sugar
¼ teaspoon salt
Black pepper to taste (optional)
1 tablespoon butter or margarine, melted

1. Preheat oven to 400°F. Line large baking sheet with foil and coat with cooking spray. Arrange vegetables in single layer on foil; coat lightly with cooking spray. Sprinkle vegetables with brown sugar, salt and pepper, if desired.

2. Bake 30 minutes. Stir gently; bake 10 to 15 minutes more or until vegetables are tender. Remove from oven. Drizzle with butter; toss to coat. *Makes 5 servings*

maple-glazed carrots & shallots

1 package (16 ounces) baby carrots
1 tablespoon margarine or butter
½ cup thinly sliced shallots
2 tablespoons reduced-fat maple-flavored pancake syrup
¼ teaspoon salt
⅛ teaspoon white pepper

1. Place carrots in medium saucepan. Add enough water to cover carrots. Bring to a boil over high heat. Reduce heat; simmer carrots over low heat 8 to 10 minutes or until carrots are tender. Drain; set aside.

2. In same saucepan, melt margarine over medium-high heat. Add shallots; cook and stir 3 to 4 minutes or until shallots are tender and beginning to brown. Add drained carrots, syrup, salt and pepper; cook and stir 1 to 2 minutes or until carrots are coated and heated through. *Makes 4 servings*

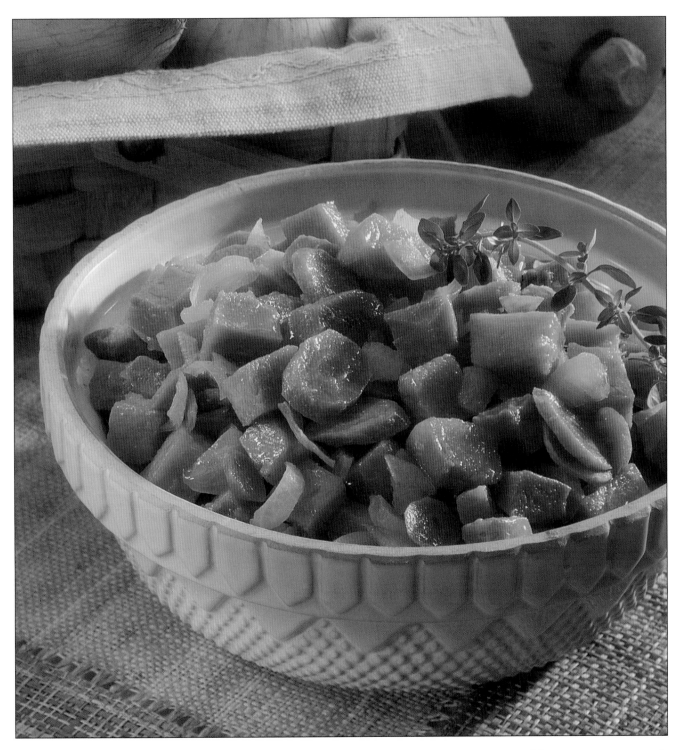

roasted butternut squash

herbed corn on the cob

nutrients per serving:

1 ear corn
Calories: 86
Carbohydrate: 14 g
Dietary Fiber: 2 g
Total Fat: 4 g
Calories From Fat: 33%
Saturated Fat: 2 g
Cholesterol: 8 mg
Sodium: 106 mg
Protein: 2 g
Exchanges: 1 Starch,
½ Fat

> 1 tablespoon butter or margarine
> 1 teaspoon mixed dried herb leaves, such as basil, oregano,
>   sage and rosemary
> ⅛ teaspoon salt
>   Black pepper
> 4 ears corn, husks removed

Microwave Directions

1. Combine butter, herbs, salt and pepper in small microwavable bowl. Microwave at MEDIUM (50% power) 30 to 45 seconds or until butter is melted.

2. With pastry brush, coat corn with butter mixture. Place corn on microwavable plate; microwave at HIGH 5 to 6 minutes. Turn corn over; microwave at HIGH 5 to 6 minutes more or until tender.   *Makes 4 servings*

marinated carrot salad

nutrients per serving:

1/12 of total recipe
Calories: 151
Carbohydrate: 16 g
Dietary Fiber: 2 g
Total Fat: 10 g
Calories From Fat: 60%
Saturated Fat: 1 g
Cholesterol: 0 mg
Sodium: 399 mg
Protein: 2 g
Exchanges: 3 Vegetable,
2 Fat

> 2 pounds carrots, sliced, or small carrots
> 1 can (10¾ ounces) tomato soup
> 1 cup EQUAL® SPOONFUL*
> 1 medium onion, chopped
> 1 green bell pepper, chopped
> ¾ cup wine vinegar
> ½ cup vegetable oil or olive oil
> 1 teaspoon Worcestershire sauce
> 1 teaspoon salt
> 1 teaspoon ground black pepper
> 1 teaspoon Dijon mustard

*May substitute 24 packets Equal® sweetener.

• Boil carrots until tender; drain.

• Combine remaining ingredients in small bowl. Pour over carrots; mix well.

• Refrigerate in covered container at least 12 hours.   *Makes 12 servings*

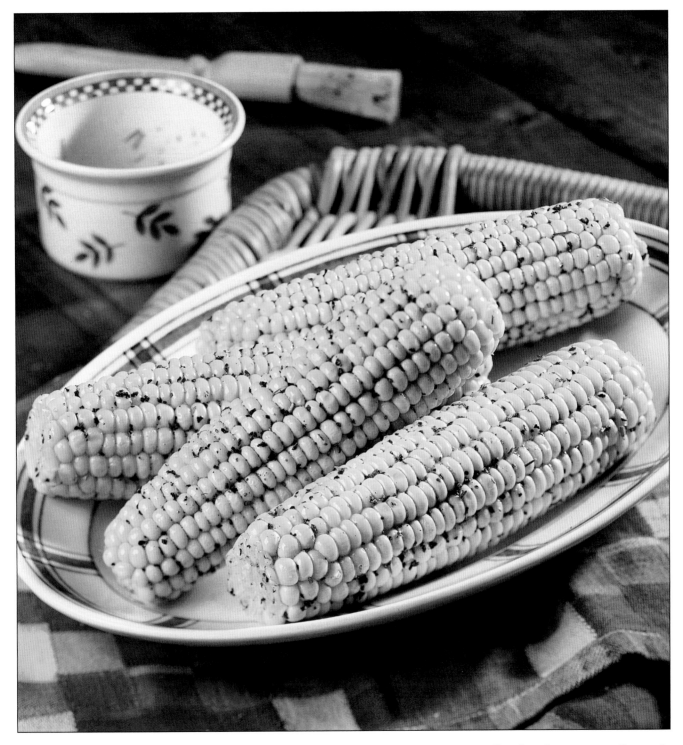

herbed corn on the cob

pepper and squash gratin

12 ounces russet potato, unpeeled
8 ounces yellow summer squash, thinly sliced
8 ounces zucchini, thinly sliced
2 cups frozen pepper stir-fry blend, thawed
1 teaspoon dried oregano leaves
½ teaspoon salt
Black pepper
½ cup grated Parmesan cheese or shredded reduced-fat sharp Cheddar cheese
1 tablespoon butter or margarine, cut into 8 pieces

1. Preheat oven to 375°F. Spray 12×8-inch glass baking dish with nonstick cooking spray. Pierce potato several times with fork. Microwave at HIGH 3 minutes. Cut potato into thin slices.

2. Layer half of potato slices, yellow squash, zucchini, pepper stir-fry blend, oregano, salt, black pepper and cheese in prepared baking dish. Repeat layers. Top with butter. Cover tightly with foil; bake 25 minutes or until vegetables are just tender. Remove foil; bake 10 minutes more or until lightly browned. *Makes 8 servings*

black-eyed peas

1 bag (1 pound) dried black-eyed peas, soaked overnight, drained
1½ cups diced onion
2 shallots, finely chopped
⅓ medium green bell pepper, cored, seeded and chopped
¼ cup vegetable oil
1 teaspoon *each* salt and black pepper
3 to 4 cups water

1. Place soaked black-eyed peas in large stockpot or Dutch oven. Add onion, shallots and bell pepper. Cover; let stand 20 minutes. Add oil, salt and black pepper; stir. Cover; let stand 10 to 15 minutes. Add enough water to cover peas by 1 inch. Bring to a boil. Lower heat; simmer, covered, 50 to 60 minutes or until tender.

2. Before serving, remove ½ cup cooked peas; mash. Return mashed peas to stockpot; stir until slightly thickened. *Makes 10 servings*

pepper and squash gratin

sweet and sour carrots

2 cups carrot slices, ¼ inch thick
½ cup celery slices, ½ inch thick
1 can (8 ounces) pineapple tidbits (drain and reserve juice)
1 tablespoon vinegar
2 teaspoons cornstarch
1 teaspoon light soy sauce
⅛ teaspoon salt
2 tablespoons stick butter or margarine
¼ cup sliced green onions
¼ cup EQUAL® SPOONFUL*

May substitute 6 packets Equal® sweetener.

• Cook carrots and celery in medium saucepan in small amount of water about 8 minutes or until tender. Drain and set aside.

• Add enough water to reserved pineapple juice to make ½ cup liquid. Stir in vinegar, cornstarch, soy sauce and salt. Cook in medium saucepan until liquid thickens.

• Add butter, drained pineapple and green onions; cook and stir until heated through. Add drained carrots and celery; cook about 2 minutes or until heated through. Stir in Equal® Spoonful. *Makes 6 servings*

tip

About 4 carrots yield 2 cups carrot slices.

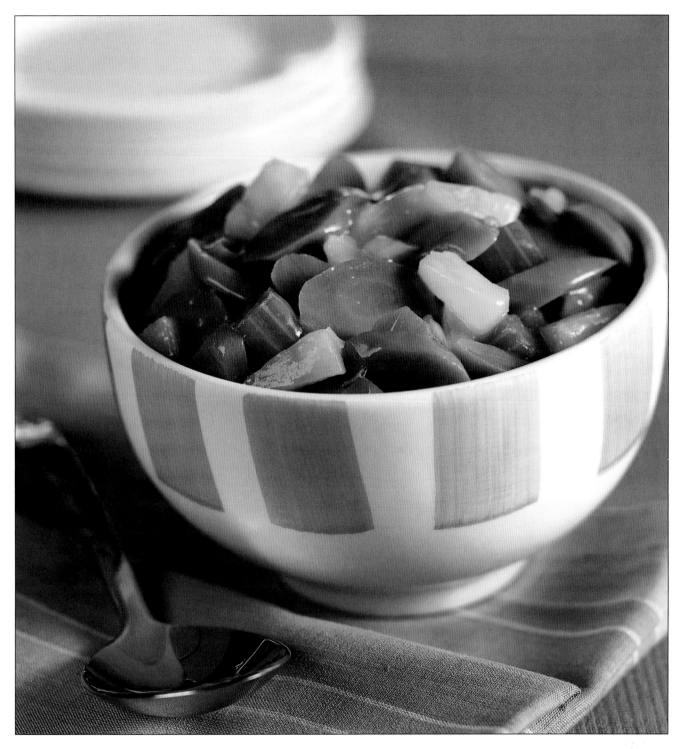

sweet and sour carrots

light lemon cauliflower

nutrients per serving:

about ⅔ cup cauliflower with 1½ tablespoons sauce and 2 teaspoons cheese
Calories: 53
Carbohydrate: 6 g
Dietary Fiber: 3 g
Total Fat: 2 g
Calories From Fat: 33%
Saturated Fat: 1 g
Cholesterol: 3 mg
Sodium: 116 mg
Protein: 4 g

Exchanges: 1 Vegetable, ½ Fat

¼ **cup chopped fresh parsley, divided**
½ **teaspoon grated lemon peel**
6 **cups (about 1½ pounds) cauliflower florets**
1 **tablespoon reduced-fat margarine**
3 **cloves garlic, minced**
2 **tablespoons fresh lemon juice**
¼ **cup shredded Parmesan cheese**

1. Place 1 tablespoon parsley, lemon peel and about 1 inch water in large saucepan. Place cauliflower in steamer basket; place in saucepan. Bring water to a boil over medium heat. Cover; steam 14 to 16 minutes or until cauliflower is crisp-tender. Remove to large bowl; keep warm. Reserve ½ cup hot liquid.

2. Heat margarine in small saucepan over medium heat. Add garlic; cook and stir 2 to 3 minutes or until soft. Stir in lemon juice and reserved liquid.

3. Spoon lemon sauce over cauliflower. Sprinkle with remaining 3 tablespoons parsley and cheese before serving. Garnish with lemon slices, if desired.

Makes 6 servings

vegetable confetti rice

nutrients per serving:

½ cup vegetable confetti rice
Calories: 90
Carbohydrate: 14 g
Dietary Fiber: 2 g
Total Fat: 2 g
Calories From Fat: 22%
Saturated Fat: <1 g
Cholesterol: 5 mg
Sodium: 103 mg
Protein: 4 g

Exchanges: ½ Starch, 1 Vegetable, ½ Lean Meat

1 **tablespoon vegetable oil**
1 **cup finely chopped celery**
½ **cup uncooked long-grain white rice**
½ **cup bottled roasted sweet red peppers, diced**
1 **can (14½ ounces) fat-free reduced-sodium chicken broth**
2 **packages (10 ounces each) mixed broccoli-cauliflower florets, cut into equal-size pieces**

1. Heat oil in large nonstick skillet over medium heat. Add celery; cook, stirring occasionally, about 5 to 6 minutes or until crisp-tender. Add rice; cook and stir about 3 to 4 minutes or until rice is opaque. Add diced red peppers; stir to combine. Add broth. Cover; simmer about 12 minutes or until rice is just cooked through.

2. Add broccoli-cauliflower florets. Cover; cook about 10 minutes or until vegetables are tender. Add water, if necessary, to prevent burning. Combine vegetables and rice before serving.

Makes 8 servings

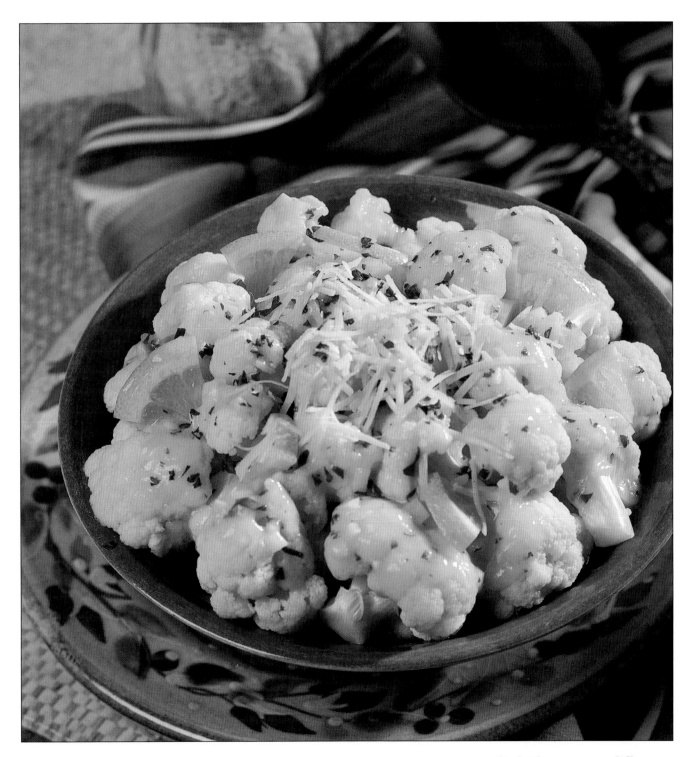

light lemon cauliflower

mashed sweet potatoes & parsnips

        2 large sweet potatoes (about 1¼ pounds), peeled and cut
            into 1-inch pieces
        2 medium parsnips (about ½ pound), peeled and cut into ½-inch slices
      ¼ cup evaporated skimmed milk
    1½ tablespoons margarine or butter
      ½ teaspoon salt
      ⅛ teaspoon ground nutmeg
      ¼ cup chopped chives or green onion tops

1. Combine sweet potatoes and parsnips in large saucepan. Cover with cold water; bring to a boil over high heat. Reduce heat; simmer, uncovered, 15 minutes or until vegetables are tender.

2. Drain vegetables; return to pan. Add milk, margarine, salt and nutmeg. Mash potato mixture over low heat to desired consistency. Stir in chives.

Makes 6 servings

nutrients per serving:

½ cup
Calories: 142
Carbohydrate: 27 g
Dietary Fiber: 4 g
Total Fat: 3 g
Calories From Fat: 19%
Saturated Fat: 1 g
Cholesterol: <1 mg
Sodium: 251 mg
Protein: 3 g
Exchanges: 1½ Starch, ½ Vegetable, ½ Fat

brussels sprouts with lemon-dill glaze

      1 pound brussels sprouts*
      2 teaspoons cornstarch
      ½ teaspoon dried dill weed
      ½ cup fat-free reduced-sodium chicken broth
      3 tablespoons lemon juice
      ½ teaspoon grated lemon peel

Or, substitute 1 package (10 ounces) frozen brussels sprouts for fresh brussels sprouts. Cook according to package directions; drain.

1. Trim brussels sprouts. Cut an "X" in stem ends. Bring 1 cup water to a boil in large saucepan over high heat. Add brussels sprouts; return to a boil. Reduce heat to medium-low. Simmer, covered, 10 minutes or just until tender. Drain well; return to pan. Set aside.

2. Meanwhile, combine cornstarch and dill weed in small saucepan. Blend in chicken broth and lemon juice until smooth. Stir in lemon peel. Cook and stir over medium heat 5 minutes or until mixture boils and thickens. Cook and stir 1 minute more. Pour glaze over brussels sprouts; toss gently to coat. Serve hot.

Makes 4 servings

nutrients per serving:

¼ of total recipe
Calories: 58
Carbohydrate: 13 g
Dietary Fiber: 5 g
Total Fat: 1 g
Calories From Fat: 9%
Saturated Fat: <1 g
Cholesterol: 0 mg
Sodium: 31 mg
Protein: 3 g
Exchanges: 2 Vegetable

mashed sweet potatoes & parsnips

vegetables with spinach fettuccine

nutrients per serving:

⅙ of total recipe
Calories: 82
Carbohydrate: 13 g
Dietary Fiber: 1 g
Total Fat: 3 g
Calories From Fat: 30%
Saturated Fat: <1 g
Cholesterol: 3 mg
Sodium: 101 mg
Protein: 3 g

Exchanges: ½ Starch, 1 Vegetable, ½ Fat

6 solid-pack sun-dried tomatoes
3 ounces uncooked spinach florentine fettuccine or spinach fettuccine
1 tablespoon olive oil
¼ cup chopped onion
¼ cup sliced red bell pepper
1 clove garlic, minced
½ cup sliced mushrooms
½ cup coarsely chopped fresh spinach
¼ teaspoon salt
¼ teaspoon ground nutmeg
⅛ teaspoon black pepper

1. Place sun-dried tomatoes in small bowl; pour boiling water over tomatoes to cover. Let stand 10 to 15 minutes or until tomatoes are tender. Drain tomatoes; discard liquid. Cut tomatoes into strips.

2. Cook pasta according to package directions, omitting salt. Drain.

3. Heat oil in large nonstick skillet over medium heat until hot. Add onion, bell pepper and garlic; cook and stir 3 minutes or until vegetables are crisp-tender. Add mushrooms and spinach; cook and stir 1 minute. Add sun-dried tomatoes, pasta, salt, nutmeg and black pepper; cook and stir 1 to 2 minutes or until heated through. Garnish as desired.

Makes 6 servings

marinated beet salad

nutrients per serving:

about ½ cup beets
Calories: 40
Carbohydrate: 10 g
Dietary Fiber: 1 g
Total Fat: 0 g
Calories From Fat: 0%
Saturated Fat: 0 g
Cholesterol: 0 mg
Sodium: 22 mg
Protein: 1 g

Exchanges: 2 Vegetable

2 cans (15 ounces each) small, whole or sliced beets
½ cup white vinegar
¾ to 1 cup EQUAL® SPOONFUL*

May substitute 18 to 24 packets Equal® sweetener.

• Combine beets, beet juice, vinegar and Equal® Spoonful in medium bowl; cover tightly.

• Chill at least 8 hours before serving. Drain before serving.

Makes 8 servings

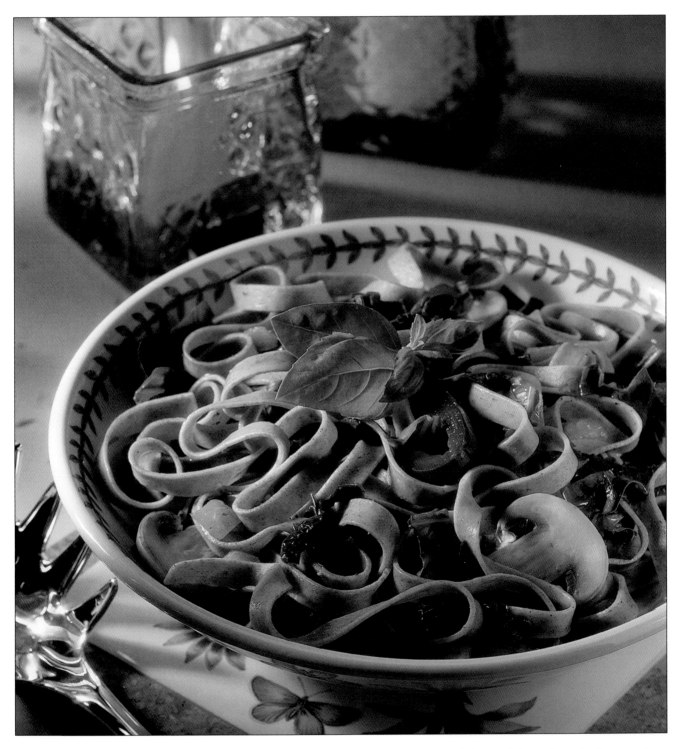

vegetables with spinach fettuccine

curried rice & green beans

nutrients per serving:

½ cup
Calories: 120
Carbohydrate: 15 g
Dietary Fiber: 1 g
Total Fat: 3 g
Calories From Fat: 25%
Saturated Fat: 1 g
Cholesterol: 14 mg
Sodium: 312 mg
Protein: 7 g

Exchanges: 1 Starch, 1 Lean Meat

    2 teaspoons vegetable oil
    2 cups sliced mushrooms
    1 clove garlic, minced
 ½ teaspoon curry powder
 ¼ teaspoon cumin seed (optional)
    1 cup fat-free reduced-sodium chicken broth
    1 cup fresh sliced green beans or frozen cut green beans
 ½ cup uncooked long-grain white rice
    4 slices Canadian bacon, cut into short thin strips
 ¼ teaspoon black pepper

1. Heat oil in small saucepan. Add mushrooms and garlic; cook and stir over medium-low heat about 5 minutes. Add curry powder and cumin seed, if desired; cook and stir 30 seconds.

2. Add chicken broth; bring to a boil. Stir in green beans and rice. Reduce heat to low. Cover; simmer about 18 minutes or until rice is tender and liquid is absorbed. Stir in Canadian bacon and pepper. Heat just until bacon is hot. *Makes 6 servings*

sweet potato puffs

nutrients per serving:

1 puff
Calories: 103
Carbohydrate: 19 g
Dietary Fiber: 2 g
Total Fat: 3 g
Calories From Fat: 21%
Saturated Fat: <1 g
Cholesterol: 21 mg
Sodium: 14 mg
Protein: 2 g

Exchanges: 1 Starch, 1 Vegetable, ½ Fat

    2 pounds sweet potatoes
 ⅓ cup orange juice
    1 egg, beaten
    1 tablespoon grated orange peel
 ½ teaspoon ground nutmeg
 ¼ cup chopped pecans

1. Peel sweet potatoes; cut into 1-inch pieces. Place potatoes in medium saucepan; add enough water to cover. Bring to a boil over medium-high heat. Cook 10 to 15 minutes or until tender. Drain potatoes; place in large bowl. Mash until smooth. Add orange juice, egg, orange peel and nutmeg; mix well.

2. Preheat oven to 375°F. Spray baking sheet with nonstick cooking spray. Spoon potato mixture into 10 mounds on prepared baking sheet. Sprinkle pecans over tops of mounds. Bake 30 minutes or until centers are hot. *Makes 10 servings*

curried rice & green beans

nutrients per serving:

about 1 cup
Calories: 91
Carbohydrate: 10 g
Dietary Fiber: 4 g
Total Fat: 3 g
Calories From Fat: 30%
Saturated Fat: 1 g
Cholesterol: 3 mg
Sodium: 188 mg
Protein: 7 g

Exchanges: ½ Starch, 1 Vegetable, ½ Fat

creamed spinach

3 cups water
2 bags (10 ounces each) washed, stemmed and chopped fresh spinach
2 teaspoons margarine
2 tablespoons all-purpose flour
1 cup fat-free (skim) milk
2 tablespoons grated Parmesan cheese
⅛ teaspoon white pepper
Ground nutmeg

1. Bring water to a boil. Add spinach. Reduce heat; simmer, covered, about 5 minutes or until spinach is wilted. Drain well; set aside.

2. Melt margarine in small saucepan over medium-low heat. Stir in flour; cook over medium-low heat 1 minute, stirring constantly. Using wire whisk, stir in milk. Bring to a boil. Cook, whisking constantly, 1 to 2 minutes or until mixture thickens. Stir in cheese and pepper.

3. Stir spinach into sauce; heat thoroughly. Spoon into serving bowl; sprinkle lightly with nutmeg. Garnish as desired.

Makes 4 servings

tip

Stem fresh spinach by first folding each leaf lengthwise in half along the stem. (The underside of the leaf should be facing you.) Pull the stem off by bringing it up towards the leaf tip.

creamed spinach

potatoes au gratin

  1 **pound baking potatoes**
  1 **tablespoon plus 1 teaspoon reduced-fat margarine**
  1 **tablespoon plus 1 teaspoon all-purpose flour**
1¼ **cups fat-free (skim) milk**
  ¼ **teaspoon ground nutmeg**
  ¼ **teaspoon paprika**
     Pinch white pepper
  ½ **cup thinly sliced red onion, divided**
  ⅓ **cup whole wheat bread crumbs**
  1 **tablespoon finely chopped red onion**
  1 **tablespoon grated Parmesan cheese**

1. Spray 4- or 6-cup casserole with nonstick cooking spray; set aside.

2. Place potatoes in large saucepan; add water to cover. Bring to a boil over high heat; boil 12 minutes or until potatoes are tender. Drain. Let potatoes stand 10 minutes or until cool enough to handle.

3. Meanwhile, melt margarine in small saucepan over medium heat. Add flour; cook and stir 3 minutes or until small clumps form. Gradually whisk in milk. Cook 8 minutes or until sauce thickens, stirring constantly. Remove saucepan from heat. Stir in nutmeg, paprika and pepper.

4. Preheat oven to 350°F. Cut potatoes into thin slices. Arrange half of potato slices in prepared casserole. Sprinkle with half of onion slices. Repeat layers. Spoon sauce over potato mixture. Combine bread crumbs, finely chopped red onion and cheese in small bowl; sprinkle evenly over sauce.

5. Bake 20 minutes. Let stand 5 minutes before serving. Garnish as desired.

Makes 4 servings

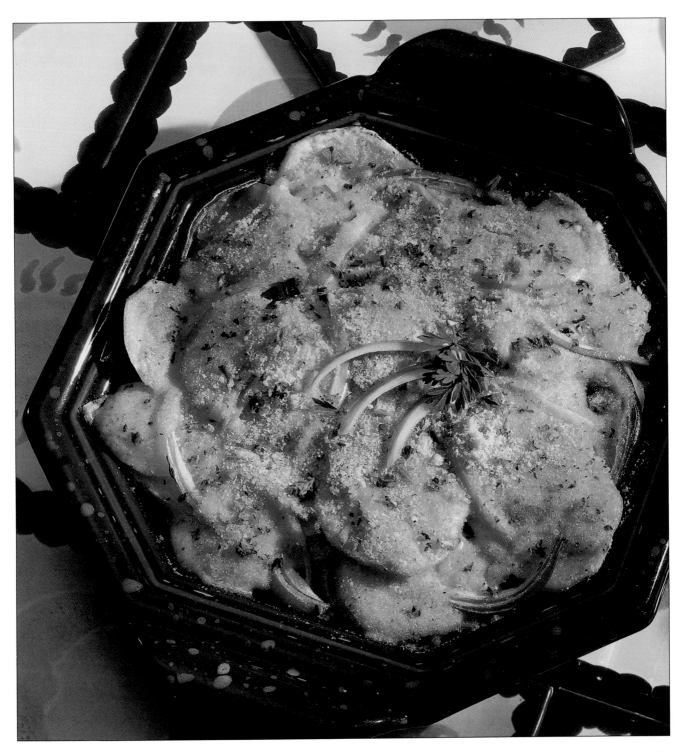

potatoes au gratin

desserts & sweets

nutrients per serving:

1 pie slice
(⅛ of total recipe)
Calories: 189
Carbohydrate: 19 g
Dietary Fiber: <1 g
Total Fat: 10 g
Calories From Fat: 48%
Saturated Fat: 4 g
Cholesterol: 61 mg
Sodium: 228 mg
Protein: 5 g
Exchanges: 1 Starch, 2 Fat

lemon meringue pie

    Pastry for single-crust 9-inch pie
2¼ **cups water**
  ½ **cup fresh lemon juice or frozen lemon juice concentrate***
  ½ **cup cornstarch**
  2 **eggs**
  2 **egg whites**
1½ **teaspoons grated lemon peel**
1½ **cups EQUAL® SPOONFUL****
  2 **tablespoons stick butter or margarine**
  1 **to 2 drops yellow food coloring (optional)**
  3 **egg whites**
  ¼ **teaspoon cream of tartar**
  ⅔ **cup EQUAL® SPOONFUL*****

*Such as Minute Maid® Premium Lemon Juice (frozen) 100% Pure Lemon Juice from Concentrate

**May substitute 36 packets Equal® sweetener.

***May substitute 16 packets Equal® sweetener.

• Roll pastry on lightly floured surface into circle 1 inch larger than inverted 9-inch pie pan. Ease pastry into pan; trim and flute edge. Pierce bottom and side of pastry with fork. Bake in preheated 425°F oven 10 to 12 minutes or until pastry is golden. Cool on wire rack.

• Combine water, lemon juice and cornstarch in medium saucepan. Bring to a boil over medium-high heat, stirring constantly; boil and stir 1 minute. Beat eggs, 2 egg whites and lemon peel in medium bowl. Mix in 1½ cups Equal® Spoonful. Stir about half of hot cornstarch mixture into egg mixture.

• Return all to saucepan. Cook and stir over low heat 1 minute. Remove from heat; stir in butter until melted. Stir in food coloring, if desired. Pour mixture into baked pie shell.

• Beat 3 egg whites in medium bowl until foamy. Add cream of tartar and beat to soft peaks. Gradually beat in ⅔ cup Equal® Spoonful, beating to stiff peaks. Spread meringue over hot lemon filling, carefully sealing to edge of crust to prevent shrinking or weeping.

• Bake pie in 425°F oven about 5 minutes or until meringue is lightly browned.

• Cool completely on wire rack before cutting. *Makes 8 servings*

lemon meringue pie

chocolate chip cookies

⅓ cup stick butter or margarine, softened
1 egg
1 teaspoon vanilla
⅓ cup EQUAL® SPOONFUL*
⅓ cup firmly packed light brown sugar
¾ cup all-purpose flour
½ teaspoon baking soda
¼ teaspoon salt
½ cup semi-sweet chocolate chips or mini chocolate chips

May substitute 8 packets Equal® sweetener.

• Beat butter with electric mixer until fluffy. Beat in egg and vanilla until blended. Mix in Equal® Spoonful and brown sugar until combined.

• Combine flour, baking soda and salt. Mix into butter mixture until well blended. Stir in chocolate chips.

• Drop dough by rounded teaspoonfuls onto ungreased baking sheet. Bake in preheated 350°F oven 8 to 10 minutes or until light golden color. Remove from baking sheet and cool completely on wire rack.   *Makes about 2 dozen cookies*

nutrients per serving:

1 cookie
Calories: 67
Carbohydrate: 8 g
Dietary Fiber: <1 g
Total Fat: 4 g
Calories From Fat: 54%
Saturated Fat: 2 g
Cholesterol: 16 mg
Sodium: 80 mg
Protein: 1 g

Exchanges: ½ Starch, 1 Fat

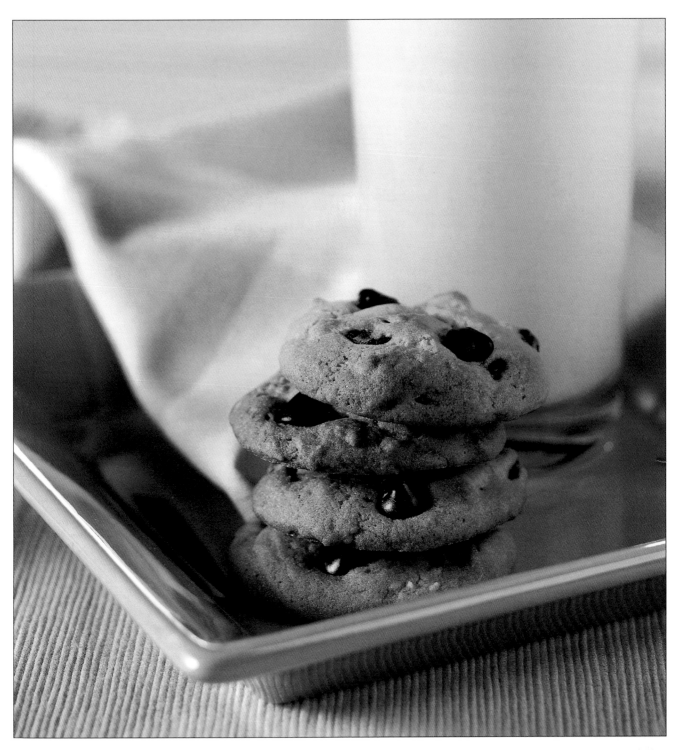

chocolate chip cookies

cranberry apple crisp

3 cups peeled and sliced apples
2 cups fresh cranberries
1 cup EQUAL® SPOONFUL*
½ cup EQUAL® SPOONFUL**
⅓ cup all-purpose flour
¼ cup chopped pecans
¼ cup stick butter or margarine, melted

May substitute 24 packets Equal® sweetener.

**May substitute 12 packets Equal® sweetener.*

● Combine apples, cranberries and 1 cup Equal® Spoonful in ungreased 10-inch pie pan.

● Combine ½ cup Equal® Spoonful, flour, pecans and butter in separate bowl. Sprinkle mixture over top of apples and cranberries.

● Bake in preheated 350°F oven about 1 hour or until bubbly and lightly browned.

Makes 8 servings

tip

This crisp is delicious served as an accompaniment to pork or poultry or with frozen yogurt as a dessert.

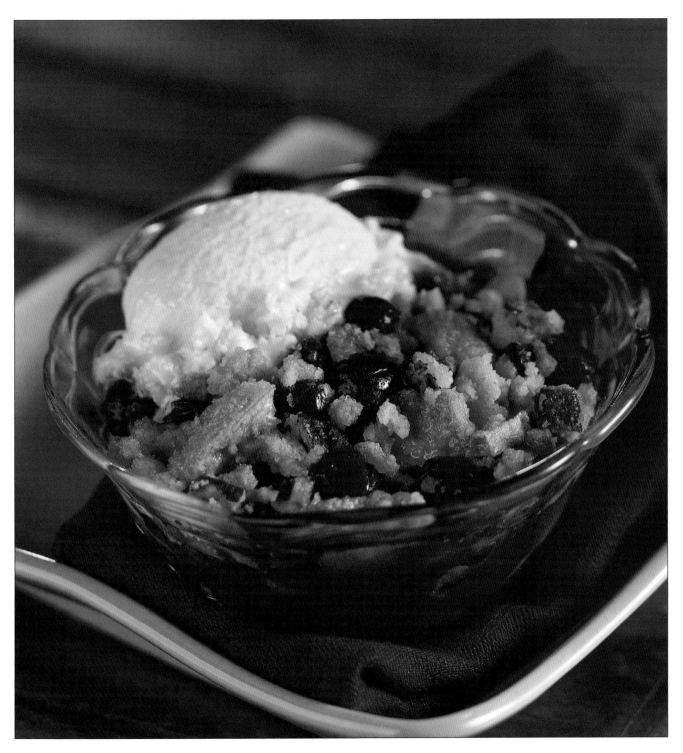

cranberry apple crisp

nutrients per serving:

1 cheesecake slice
(⅛ of total recipe)
Calories: 197
Carbohydrate: 14 g
Dietary Fiber: <1 g
Total Fat: 11 g
Calories From Fat: 50%
Saturated Fat: 8 g
Cholesterol: 58 mg
Sodium: 366 mg
Protein: 9 g
Exchanges: 1 Milk, 2 Fat

cool lime cheesecake

1 cup graham cracker crumbs
3 tablespoons stick butter or margarine, melted
2 tablespoons EQUAL® SPOONFUL*
2 packages (8 ounces each) reduced-fat cream cheese, softened
⅔ cup EQUAL® SPOONFUL**
1 egg
2 egg whites
½ teaspoon grated lime peel
3 tablespoon fresh lime juice

*May substitute 3 packets Equal® sweetener.

**May substitute 16 packets Equal® sweetener.

• Combine graham cracker crumbs, butter and 2 tablespoons Equal® Spoonful in bottom of 8-inch springform pan or 8-inch cake pan; pat evenly onto bottom and ½ inch up side of pan. Bake in preheated 325°F oven 8 minutes.

• Beat cream cheese and ⅔ cup Equal® Spoonful in medium bowl until fluffy. Beat in egg, egg whites, lime peel and juice until well blended. Pour cream cheese mixture into prepared crust.

• Bake in 325°F oven 30 to 35 minutes or until center is almost set. Cool on wire rack. Refrigerate at least 3 hours before serving. *Makes 8 servings*

nutrients per serving:

1 cake slice with
1 tablespoon plus
1 teaspoon sauce
(1/12 of total recipe)
Calories: 84
Carbohydrate: 19 g
Dietary Fiber: 1 g
Total Fat: <1 g
Calories From Fat: 3%
Saturated Fat: <1 g
Cholesterol: <1 mg
Sodium: 218 mg
Protein: 2 g
Exchanges: 1 Starch

angel food cake with blueberry yogurt sauce

½ cup frozen blueberries
Purchased small round angel food cake
½ cup vanilla nonfat yogurt
1 tablespoon granulated sugar
1 teaspoon lemon juice

Allow blueberries to thaw slightly. Cut angel food cake into 12 slices. Stir together yogurt, sugar and lemon juice in small bowl. To serve, spoon yogurt mixture and blueberries evenly over cake slices. *Makes 12 servings*

Favorite recipe from The Sugar Association, Inc.

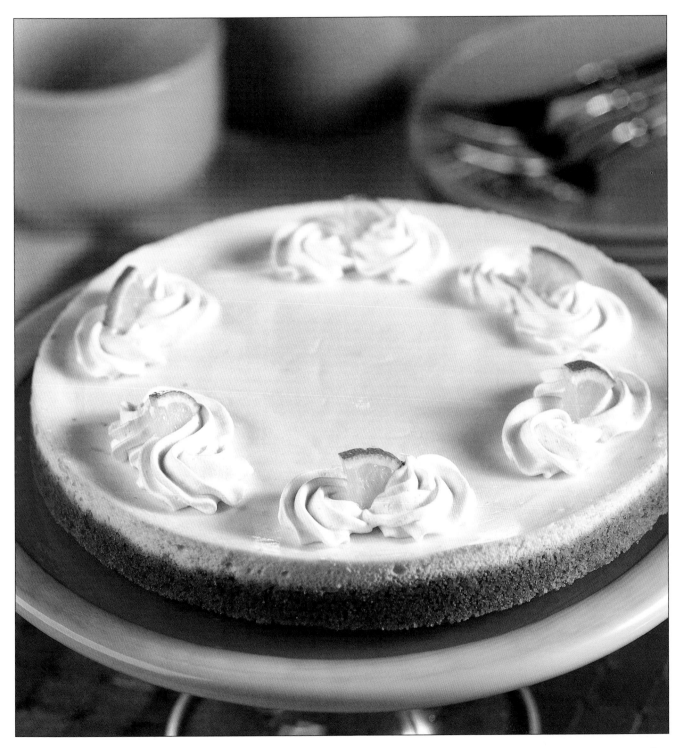

cool lime cheesecake

fresh strawberry cream pie

1 quart fresh medium strawberries
1 tablespoon EQUAL® SPOONFUL*
   Pastry for single-crust 9-inch pie, baked
1 package (8 ounces) reduced-fat cream cheese, softened
⅓ cup vanilla-flavored light nonfat yogurt
¼ cup EQUAL® SPOONFUL**
1 tablespoon lemon juice

*May substitute 1½ packets Equal® sweetener.

**May substitute 6 packets Equal® sweetener.

● Remove stems from several strawberries and slice to make 1 cup. Toss with
1 tablespoon Equal® Spoonful. Spread on bottom of baked pie shell.

● Beat cream cheese, yogurt, ¼ cup Equal® Spoonful and 1 tablespoon lemon juice
until smooth and fluffy. Spread over sliced strawberries in pie shell. Remove stems from
all but 1 large strawberry. Cut berries lengthwise in half. Place, cut side down, over
cream cheese mixture, around outer edge of pie crust, with pointed ends of berries
facing center of pie. Make several thin slits in last whole berry, starting near top and
going to pointed end. Press gently with fingers to form "fan." Place in center of pie.

● Refrigerate pie at least 4 hours before serving.   *Makes 8 servings*

tip

Unwrap 1 package (8 ounces) of cream cheese.
Place the cream cheese on a microwavable plate.
Heat at MEDIUM (50% power) 15 to 20 seconds or
just until it is softened. Allow cream cheese to stand
about 1 minute before using.

fresh strawberry cream pie

berries with banana cream

⅓ **cup reduced-fat sour cream**
½ **small ripe banana, cut into chunks**
1 **tablespoon frozen orange juice concentrate**
2 **cups sliced strawberries, blueberries, raspberries or a combination**
   Ground cinnamon or nutmeg

1. Combine sour cream, banana and juice concentrate in blender. Cover; blend until smooth.

2. Place berries in 2 serving dishes. Top with sour cream mixture. Sprinkle with cinnamon. *Makes 2 servings*

nutrients per serving:

1 cup berries with about 3 tablespoons sour cream mixture
Calories: 135
Carbohydrate: 23 g
Dietary Fiber: 4 g
Total Fat: 4 g
Calories From Fat: 25%
Saturated Fat: 3 g
Cholesterol: 13 mg
Sodium: 29 mg
Protein: 4 g

Exchanges: 1½ Fruit, 1 Fat

applesauce molasses snacking cake

1½ **cups all-purpose flour**
1 **cup whole wheat flour**
1 **teaspoon baking soda**
1 **teaspoon ground cinnamon**
¼ **teaspoon ground allspice**
1 **cup firmly packed dark brown sugar**
½ **cup FLEISCHMANN'S® Original Margarine, softened**
1¼ **cups sweetened applesauce**
½ **cup EGG BEATERS®**
⅓ **cup light molasses**
½ **cup seedless raisins**
   Powdered sugar, optional

In medium bowl, combine all-purpose flour, whole wheat flour, baking soda, cinnamon and allspice; set aside.

In large bowl, with electric mixer at medium speed, beat brown sugar and margarine until creamy. Add applesauce, Egg Beaters® and molasses; beat until smooth. Gradually add flour mixture, beating until well blended. Stir in raisins. Spread batter into ungreased 15×10×1-inch baking pan. Bake at 350°F for 20 to 25 minutes or until toothpick inserted into center comes out clean. Cool in pan on wire rack. Dust with powdered sugar before serving, if desired. Cut into 48 (2×1-inch) bars. *Makes 4 dozen bars*

Prep Time: 25 minutes
Bake Time: 25 minutes

nutrients per serving:

1 bar
Calories: 74
Carbohydrate: 14 g
Dietary Fiber: 1 g
Total Fat: 2 g
Calories From Fat: 24%
Saturated Fat: <1 g
Cholesterol: 0 mg
Sodium: 59 mg
Protein: 1 g

Exchanges: 1 Starch

berries with banana cream

bittersweet chocolate torte

nutrients per serving:

1 torte slice
(¹⁄₁₂ of total recipe)

Calories: 145
Carbohydrate: 9 g
Dietary Fiber: 2 g
Total Fat: 12 g
Calories From Fat: 74%
Saturated Fat: 7 g
Cholesterol: 36 mg
Sodium: 116 mg
Protein: 3 g

Exchanges: ½ Starch,
2 Fat

Torte
   6 tablespoons stick butter or margarine
   4 ounces unsweetened chocolate
   ⅓ cup fat-free milk
   ⅓ cup sugar-free apricot preserves or apricot spreadable fruit
   2 teaspoons instant coffee crystals
   1 egg yolk
   1 teaspoon vanilla
   1½ cups EQUAL® SPOONFUL*
   3 egg whites
   ⅛ teaspoon cream of tartar
   ¼ cup all-purpose flour
   ⅛ teaspoon salt

Rich Chocolate Glaze
   1 ounce semi-sweet chocolate
   1 tablespoon stick butter or margarine
   Whipped topping, fresh raspberries and/or fresh mint (optional)

May substitute 36 packets Equal® sweetener.

● For Torte, heat 6 tablespoons butter, 4 ounces chocolate, milk, preserves and coffee crystals in small saucepan, whisking frequently until chocolate is almost melted.

● Remove pan from heat; continue whisking until chocolate is melted and mixture is smooth. Whisk in egg yolk and vanilla; add Equal® Spoonful, whisking until smooth.

● Lightly grease bottom of 8-inch cake pan and line with parchment or waxed paper. Beat egg whites and cream of tartar to stiff peaks in large bowl. Fold chocolate mixture into egg whites; fold in combined flour and salt. Pour cake batter into pan.

● Bake in preheated 350°F oven 20 to 25 minutes or until wooden pick inserted in center comes out clean. Do not overbake. Carefully loosen side of cake from pan with small sharp knife, which will keep cake from cracking as it cools. Cool cake completely in pan on wire rack; refrigerate 1 to 2 hours or until chilled.

● For Rich Chocolate Glaze, melt 1 ounce semi-sweet chocolate and 1 tablespoon butter in small saucepan, stirring frequently.

● Remove cake from pan and place on serving plate. Pour Rich Chocolate Glaze over top of cake, letting it run down sides. Let cake stand 1 hour or until glaze is set. Garnish top with whipped topping, raspberries and mint.   *Makes 12 servings*

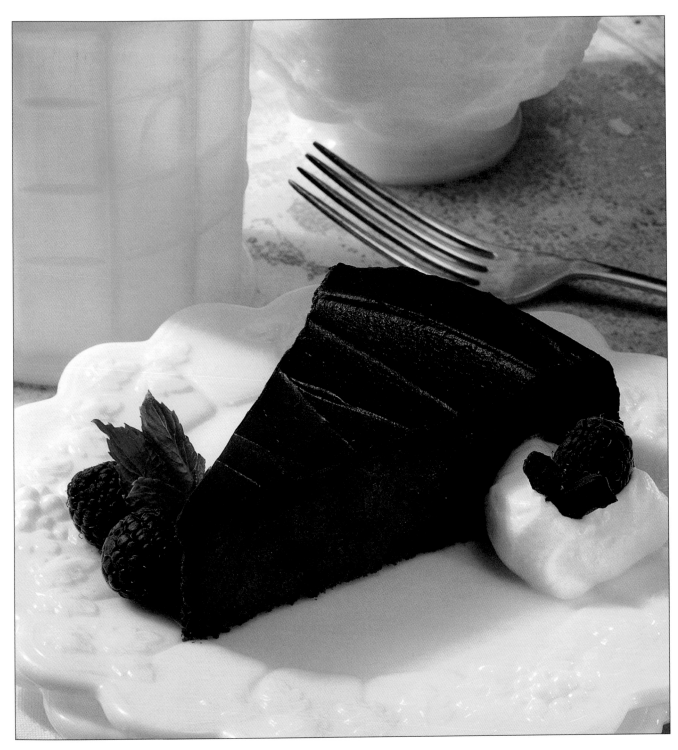

bittersweet chocolate torte

1 cheesecake slice
($\frac{1}{16}$ of total recipe)
Calories: 196
Carbohydrate: 13 g
Dietary Fiber: 1 g
Total Fat: 13 g
Calories From Fat: 60%
Saturated Fat: 7 g
Cholesterol: 62 mg
Sodium: 268 mg
Protein: 7 g

Exchanges: 1 Starch, 2½ Fat

cranberry orange cheesecake

1 ⅓ cups gingersnap crumbs
3 tablespoons EQUAL® SPOONFUL*
3 tablespoons stick butter or margarine, melted
3 packages (8 ounces each) reduced-fat cream cheese, softened
1 cup EQUAL® SPOONFUL**
2 eggs
2 egg whites
2 tablespoons cornstarch
¼ teaspoon salt
1 cup reduced-fat sour cream
2 teaspoons vanilla
1 cup chopped fresh or frozen cranberries
1 ½ teaspoons grated orange peel

*May substitute 4½ packets Equal® sweetener.

**May substitute 24 packets Equal® sweetener.

• Mix gingersnap crumbs, 3 tablespoons Equal® Spoonful and melted butter in bottom of 9-inch springform pan. Reserve 2 tablespoons crumb mixture. Pat remaining mixture evenly onto bottom of pan. Bake in preheated 325°F oven 8 minutes. Cool on wire rack.

• Beat cream cheese and 1 cup Equal® Spoonful in large bowl until fluffy; beat in eggs, egg whites, cornstarch and salt. Beat in sour cream and vanilla until blended. Gently stir in cranberries and orange peel. Pour batter into crust in pan. Sprinkle with reserved crumb mixture.

• Bake in 325°F oven 45 to 50 minutes or until center is almost set. Remove cheesecake to wire rack. Gently run metal spatula around rim of pan to loosen cake. Let cheesecake cool completely; cover and refrigerate several hours or overnight before serving. To serve, remove sides of springform pan. *Makes 16 servings*

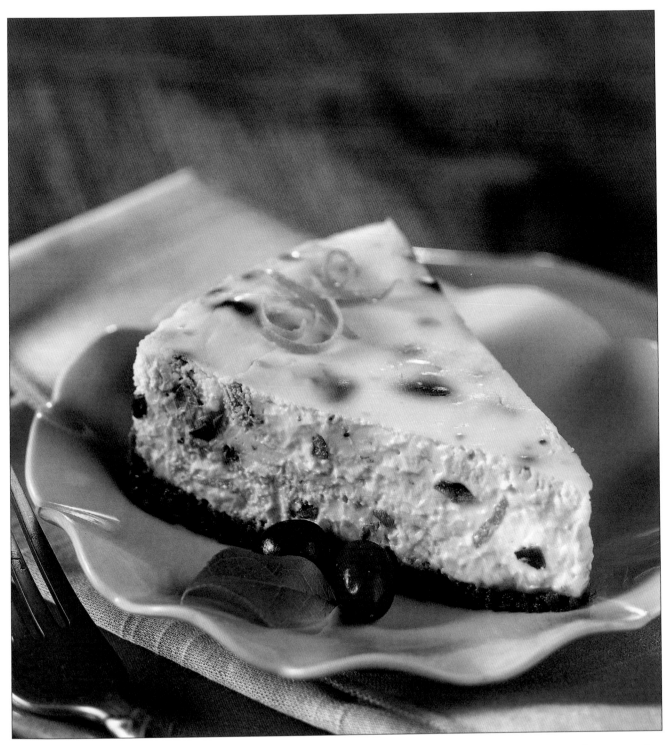

cranberry orange cheesecake

apricot biscotti

3 cups all-purpose flour
1½ teaspoons baking soda
½ teaspoon salt
⅔ cup sugar
3 eggs
1 teaspoon vanilla
½ cup chopped dried apricots*
⅓ cup sliced almonds, chopped
1 tablespoon reduced-fat (2%) milk

Other chopped dried fruits, such as dried cherries, cranberries or blueberries, can be substituted.

1. Preheat oven to 350°F. Lightly coat cookie sheet with nonstick cooking spray; set aside.

2. Combine flour, baking soda and salt in medium bowl; set aside.

3. Beat sugar, eggs and vanilla in large bowl with electric mixer at medium speed until blended. Add flour mixture; beat until well blended.

4. Stir in apricots and almonds. Turn dough out onto lightly floured work surface. Knead 4 to 6 times. Shape dough into 20-inch log; place on prepared cookie sheet. Brush dough with milk.

5. Bake 30 minutes or until firm. Remove from oven to wire rack; cool 10 minutes. Slice diagonally into 30 biscotti. Place slices on cookie sheet. Bake 10 minutes; turn and bake additional 10 minutes. Cool on wire rack. Store in airtight container.

Makes 30 servings

apricot biscotti

pear-ginger upside-down cake

2 unpeeled Bosc or Anjou pears, cored and sliced into ¼-inch-thick pieces
3 tablespoons fresh lemon juice
1 to 2 tablespoons melted butter
1 to 2 tablespoons packed brown sugar
1 cup all-purpose flour
1 teaspoon baking powder
1 teaspoon ground cinnamon
¼ teaspoon baking soda
⅛ teaspoon salt
⅓ cup fat-free (skim) milk
3 tablespoons no-sugar-added apricot fruit spread
1 egg
1 tablespoon vegetable oil
1 tablespoon minced fresh ginger

1. Preheat oven to 375°F. Spray 10-inch deep-dish pie pan with nonstick cooking spray; set aside.

2. Toss pears in lemon juice; drain. Brush butter evenly onto bottom of prepared pan; sprinkle sugar over butter. Arrange pears in pan; bake 10 minutes.

3. Meanwhile, combine flour, baking powder, cinnamon, baking soda and salt in small bowl; set aside. Combine milk, apricot spread, egg, oil and ginger in medium bowl; mix well. Add flour mixture; stir until well mixed. (Batter will be very thick.) Carefully spread batter evenly over pears to edge of pan.

4. Bake 20 to 25 minutes or until golden brown and toothpick inserted into center comes out clean.

5. Remove pan to wire rack; cool 5 minutes. Use knife to loosen cake from side of pan. Place 10-inch plate over top of pan; quickly turn over to transfer cake to plate. Place any pears left in pan on top of cake. Serve warm.

Makes 8 servings

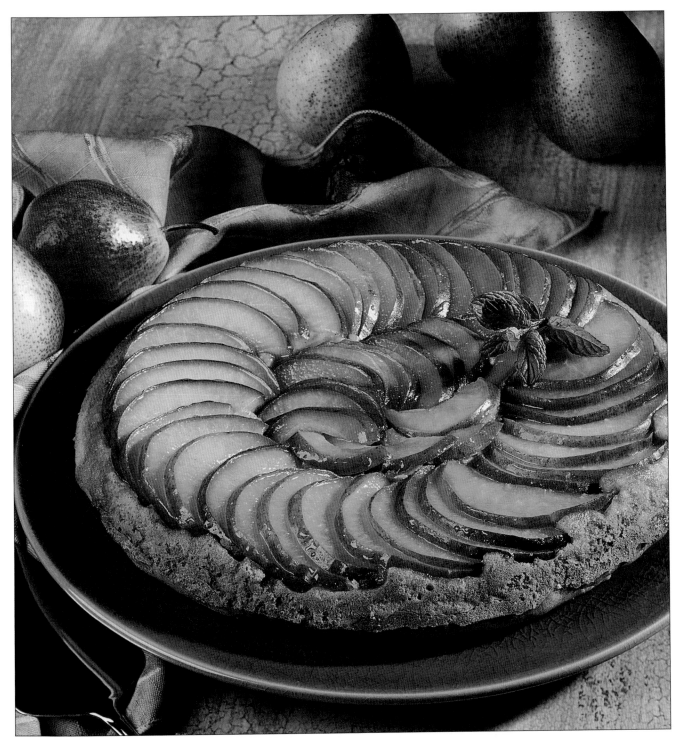

pear-ginger upside-down cake

rice pudding mexicana

1 package (4-serving size) fat-free rice pudding
1 tablespoon vanilla
¼ teaspoon ground cinnamon
Dash ground cloves
¼ cup slivered almonds
Additional ground cinnamon

1. Prepare rice pudding according to package directions.

2. Remove pudding from heat; stir in vanilla, ¼ teaspoon cinnamon and cloves. Divide evenly among 6 individual dessert dishes.

3. Top evenly with almonds and additional cinnamon. Serve warm.

Makes 6 servings

nutrients per serving:

1 dessert dish rice pudding (⅙ of total recipe)
Calories: 146
Carbohydrate: 22 g
Dietary Fiber: 1 g
Total Fat: 4 g
Calories From Fat: 27%
Saturated Fat: 1 g
Cholesterol: 6 mg
Sodium: 106 mg
Protein: 4 g
Exchanges: 1 Starch, ½ Milk, ½ Fat

banana pistachio pie

¾ cup cinnamon graham cracker crumbs
2 tablespoons reduced-fat margarine, melted
2 packages (4-serving size each) fat-free sugar-free instant pistachio pudding and pie filling mix
2½ cups fat-free (skim) milk
1 large ripe banana, sliced
¼ teaspoon ground cinnamon
1 cup thawed frozen reduced-fat nondairy whipped topping
Additional thawed frozen reduced-fat nondairy whipped topping (optional)

1. Combine graham cracker crumbs and margarine in small bowl; stir with fork until crumbly. Press crumb mixture onto bottom of 9-inch pie plate.

2. Prepare pudding mix according to manufacturer's pie directions, using 2½ cups milk. Gently stir in banana and cinnamon; fold in 1 cup whipped topping. Pour into prepared crust. Refrigerate at least 1 hour. Top with additional whipped topping before serving, if desired.

Makes 8 servings

nutrients per serving:

1 pie slice (⅛ of total recipe)
Calories: 143
Carbohydrate: 22 g
Dietary Fiber: 1 g
Total Fat: 4 g
Calories From Fat: 24%
Saturated Fat: 1 g
Cholesterol: 2 mg
Sodium: 450 mg
Protein: 3 g
Exchanges: 1½ Starch, 1 Fat

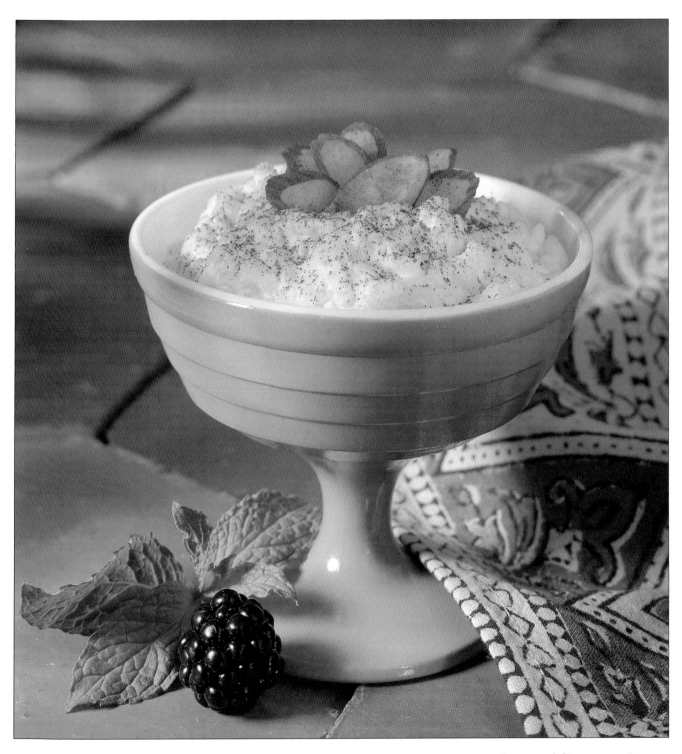

rice pudding mexicana

nutrients per serving:

1 tart slice
(⅛ of total recipe)
Calories: 139
Carbohydrate: 25 g
Dietary Fiber: 2 g
Total Fat: 4 g
Calories From Fat: 25%
Saturated Fat: 4 g
Cholesterol: 0 mg
Sodium: 59 mg
Protein: 2 g

Exchanges: 1 Starch,
½ Fruit, ½ Fat

tropical fruit coconut tart

1 cup cornflakes, crushed
1 can (3½ ounces) sweetened flaked coconut
2 egg whites
1 can (15¼ ounces) pineapple chunks in juice, undrained
2 teaspoons cornstarch
2 packets sugar substitute *or* equivalent of 4 teaspoons sugar
1 teaspoon coconut extract (optional)
1 mango, peeled and thinly sliced
1 medium banana, thinly sliced

1. Preheat oven to 425°F. Coat 9-inch springform pan with nonstick cooking spray; set aside.

2. Combine cornflakes, coconut and egg whites in medium bowl; toss gently to blend. Place mixture in prepared pan; press firmly to cover bottom and ½ inch up side of pan. Bake 8 minutes or until edge begins to brown. Cool completely on wire rack.

3. Drain pineapple, reserving juice. Combine pineapple juice and cornstarch in small saucepan; stir until cornstarch is dissolved. Bring to a boil over high heat. Continue boiling 1 minute, stirring constantly. Remove from heat; cool completely. Stir in sugar substitute and coconut extract, if desired.

4. Combine pineapple, mango slices and banana slices in medium bowl. Spoon over baked crust; drizzle with pineapple juice mixture. Cover with plastic wrap; refrigerate 2 hours. Garnish with pineapple leaves, if desired. *Makes 8 servings*

Note: The crust may be made 24 hours in advance, if desired.

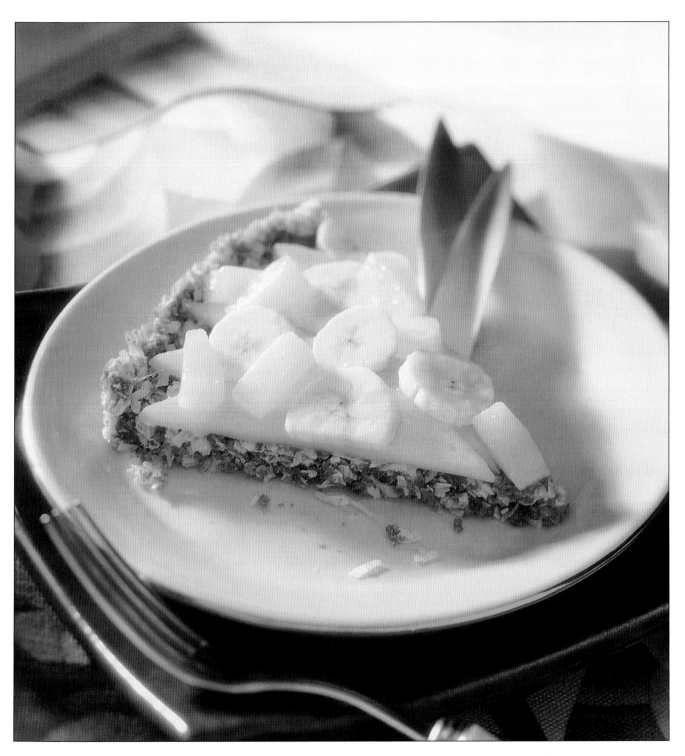

tropical fruit coconut tart

nutrients per serving:

1 cheesecake slice (1/16 of total recipe)
Calories: 152
Carbohydrate: 11 g
Dietary Fiber: 1 g
Total Fat: 10 g
Calories From Fat: 59%
Saturated Fat: 6 g
Cholesterol: 31 mg
Sodium: 158 mg
Protein: 6 g
Exchanges: 1 Milk, 2 Fat

orange chiffon cheesecake

Crust
   1 cup graham cracker crumbs
   3 tablespoons EQUAL® SPOONFUL*
   3 tablespoons stick butter or margarine, melted

Filling
   1 cup orange juice
   1 envelope unflavored gelatin
   2 packages (8 ounces each) reduced-fat cream cheese, softened
   1 cup part-skim ricotta cheese
   ¾ cup EQUAL® SPOONFUL**
   1 teaspoon orange extract (optional)
   2 cups light whipped topping
   1 can (11 ounces) mandarin oranges, drained, coarsely chopped

*May substitute 4½ packets Equal® sweetener.

**May substitute 18 packets Equal® sweetener.

• For crust, combine all ingredients. Press onto bottom of 9-inch springform pan. Bake in preheated 350°F oven 10 minutes. Remove from oven and cool on wire rack while preparing filling.

• For filling, pour orange juice into small saucepan. Sprinkle gelatin over orange juice and let soften 1 minute. Heat over low heat, stirring constantly until gelatin is completely dissolved. Remove from heat; set aside. Beat cream cheese and ricotta cheese in medium-size bowl with electric mixer until smooth and fluffy. Mix in Equal® Spoonful and orange extract until combined. Stir in gelatin mixture. Place cheese mixture in refrigerator or freezer 20 to 30 minutes to thicken slightly. Fold in whipped topping and orange pieces. Spread evenly over baked crust.

• Refrigerate several hours or overnight. To serve, place springform pan on serving plate; remove sides of pan. Garnish with additional orange slices and whipped topping, if desired.   *Makes 16 servings*

METRIC CONVERSION CHART

VOLUME MEASUREMENTS (dry)

1/8 teaspoon = 0.5 mL
1/4 teaspoon = 1 mL
1/2 teaspoon = 2 mL
3/4 teaspoon = 4 mL
1 teaspoon = 5 mL
1 tablespoon = 15 mL
2 tablespoons = 30 mL
1/4 cup = 60 mL
1/3 cup = 75 mL
1/2 cup = 125 mL
2/3 cup = 150 mL
3/4 cup = 175 mL
1 cup = 250 mL
2 cups = 1 pint = 500 mL
3 cups = 750 mL
4 cups = 1 quart = 1 L

VOLUME MEASUREMENTS (fluid)

1 fluid ounce (2 tablespoons) = 30 mL
4 fluid ounces (1/2 cup) = 125 mL
8 fluid ounces (1 cup) = 250 mL
12 fluid ounces (1 1/2 cups) = 375 mL
16 fluid ounces (2 cups) = 500 mL

WEIGHTS (mass)

1/2 ounce = 15 g
1 ounce = 30 g
3 ounces = 90 g
4 ounces = 120 g
8 ounces = 225 g
10 ounces = 285 g
12 ounces = 360 g
16 ounces = 1 pound = 450 g

DIMENSIONS

1/16 inch = 2 mm
1/8 inch = 3 mm
1/4 inch = 6 mm
1/2 inch = 1.5 cm
3/4 inch = 2 cm
1 inch = 2.5 cm

OVEN TEMPERATURES

250°F = 120°C
275°F = 140°C
300°F = 150°C
325°F = 160°C
350°F = 180°C
375°F = 190°C
400°F = 200°C
425°F = 220°C
450°F = 230°C

BAKING PAN SIZES

Utensil	Size in Inches/Quarts	Metric Volume	Size in Centimeters
Baking or Cake Pan (square or rectangular)	8×8×2	2 L	20×20×5
	9×9×2	2.5 L	23×23×5
	12×8×2	3 L	30×20×5
	13×9×2	3.5 L	33×23×5
Loaf Pan	8×4×3	1.5 L	20×10×7
	9×5×3	2 L	23×13×7
Round Layer Cake Pan	8×1½	1.2 L	20×4
	9×1½	1.5 L	23×4
Pie Plate	8×1¼	750 mL	20×3
	9×1¼	1 L	23×3
Baking Dish or Casserole	1 quart	1 L	—
	1½ quart	1.5 L	—
	2 quart	2 L	—

acknowledgments

The publisher would like to thank the companies and organizations listed below for the use of their recipes and photographs in this publication.

Egg Beaters®
Equal® sweetener
Mrs. Dash®
The Sugar Association, Inc.
USA Rice

recipe index

316 • Recipe Index

R

Radishes: Teriyaki Salmon with Asian Slaw, 234

Raisins
Applesauce Molasses Snacking Cake, 294
Pork Roast with Dried Cranberries and Apricots, 244

Raspberries
Berries with Banana Cream, 294
Raspberry Mango Salad, 212

Rice
Curried Rice & Green Beans, 278
Rice Pudding Mexicana, 304
Shrimp Étouffée, 220
Vegetable Confetti Rice, 272
Rice Bran Buttermilk Pancakes, 156
Rice Pudding Mexicana, 304
Roasted Butternut Squash, 264
Roasted Eggplant Rolls, 196
Roasted Red Pepper & Tomato Casserole, 258
Rock 'n' Rollers, 194

Rolls: California Rolls, 188

S

Salads
Chicken and Spinach Salad, 224
Mandarin Turkey Salad with Buttermilk-Herb Dressing, 204
Marinated Beet Salad, 276
Marinated Carrot Salad, 266
Raspberry Mango Salad, 212
Salmon Pasta Salad, 226
Sunburst Chicken Salad, 222

Salmon
Salmon Pasta Salad, 226
Teriyaki Salmon with Asian Slaw, 234
Salmon Pasta Salad, 226

Salmon, Smoked (see also Lox): Smoked Salmon Appetizers, 198

Salsa
Avocado Salsa, 200
Cheesy Potato Skin Appetizers, 185
Super Nachos, 198
Zesty Pico de Gallo, 180

Sandwiches
Broiled Turkey Burgers, 228
Garden Tuna Salad, 206
Grilled Mozzarella & Roasted Red Pepper Sandwich, 222
Grilled Portobello Open-Faced Sandwich, 224
Huevos Ranchwich, 208
Stuffed Party Baguette, 190
Tangy Italian Chicken Sandwiches, 206
Turkey Sandwiches with Roasted Bell Peppers, 218
Sassy Chicken & Peppers, 248

Sausage, Pork: Brunch Strata, 174

Scallops: Broccoli, Scallop and Linguine Toss, 246
Scrambled Egg Burritos, 176
Señor Nacho Dip, 188

Sesame Oil: Portobello Mushrooms Sesame, 186

Shallots
Black-Eyed Peas, 268
Maple-Glazed Carrots & Shallots, 264

Shrimp: Shrimp Étouffée, 220
Smoked Salmon Appetizers, 198
Snackin' Cinnamon Popcorn, 192

Snow Peas
Eggs Primavera, 170
Teriyaki Salmon with Asian Slaw, 234

Soups & Stews
Black and White Chili, 228
Chunky Chicken Stew, 214
Shrimp Étouffée, 220

Soups & Stews (continued)
Tuscan Chicken with White Beans, 214
Vegetable-Chicken Noodle Soup, 212

Sour Cream
Berries with Banana Cream, 294
Blueberry-Sour Cream Corn Muffins, 164
Cranberry Orange Cheesecake, 298

Spaghetti Sauce: Roasted Eggplant Rolls, 196
Spicy Mexican Frittata, 178
Spicy Mustard Dip, 188
Spicy Orange Chicken Kabob Appetizers, 192
Spicy Vegetable Quesadillas, 200

Spinach
California Rolls, 188
Cannelloni with Tomato-Eggplant Sauce, 250
Chicken and Spinach Salad, 224
Chicken with Spinach and Celery Hash, 254
Creamed Spinach, 280
Fresh Vegetable Lasagna, 238
Roasted Eggplant Rolls, 196
Rock 'n' Rollers, 194
Vegetables with Spinach Fettuccine, 276

Sprouts, Alfalfa: California Rolls, 188

Squash (see also Squash, Summer; Zucchini): Roasted Butternut Squash, 264

Squash, Summer (see also Zucchini)
Eggs Primavera, 170
Pepper and Squash Gratin, 268

Stir-Fry: Sweet and Sour Stir-Fry, 256

Strata: Brunch Strata, 174

general index